What *Killed* Sally

The tragic yet informative safety guide for
knowing your way around

PSL Ranch, Menard County, Texas

SLIM AND CASSY

ISBN 978-1-64300-745-8 (Paperback)
ISBN 978-1-64300-746-5 (Digital)

Covenant Books, Inc.
11661 Hwy 707
Murrells Inlet, SC 29576
www.covenantbooks.com

Contents

Prologue

The youth organization, Green Tree Campers of America (GTCA), loves to spend time in the wilderness educating their young, mostly city-born members, in the ways of nature. Spending time outdoors on educational adventures with their fellow GTCA members is by far their favorite activity.

PSL Ranch allows these young adventurers to camp on our remote patch of wilderness to observe the local fauna, flora, and rock formations that were created a millennium ago. Although this Menard County ranchland is beautiful and full of interesting wildlife, it can also be quite dangerous for the unprepared and those not knowledgeable of local conditions. Due to a *few* incidents that have occurred during camping expeditions by the GTCA (thirty-nine that we know of), PSL ranch hands decided to put together this informational guide to give visitors an educational approach to safety and possibly avoid an unpleasant injury, maiming, or death while providing facts about the local environment and wildlife.

Each incident will be discussed in varying amounts of detail; gaps in knowledge will be filled in with good old-fashioned Texas bullshit. It should be noted that there are not thirty-nine bodies buried or dispersed on PSL ranch. The actual number is believed to be much lower as coyotes and other large predators tend to carry them away.

Now sit back in your favorite seat and enjoy this educational adventure!

Introduction

When the owners first laid eyes on this ranchland, "What a P.S.L.!" Rolled off the lips of one, hence the name PSL Ranch. Located on an isolated plat off a cattle lane near Menard Texas (the closest large city), this ranchland has been relatively untouched by human activity as it sits at the very end of the road—quite literally. Not having modern conveniences such as electricity and drinkable water until recently[1], this remote piece of God's country was and is overrun with wildlife, cactus, mesquite trees, and live oak; providing the perfect get-a-way for dedicated campers. It should also be noted that there is *no* connectivity at PSL Ranch; no phone lines, no cell service, and no Internet. This has been known to be the demise of several millennials like Sally.

Why Sally?

What did Sally ever do to you?

These questions are often asked of ranch hands by visitors or during interrogations by law enforcement officers and federal investigators following an incident. The simple answer is, "Why *not* Sally?" After all, it's not PSL Ranch's fault an unusually high percentage of GTCA members have the name Sally. It does seem a bit odd though that those named Sally appear to have a lower than normal aptitude for living outdoors.

Some would even say, "She really sucks at it!" But if you're named Sally, don't fret, you are still welcome at PSL Ranch. We've

---

[1] The term *Drinkable* is a word used liberally on PSL Ranch and is often debated. For instance, should you be able to see through a glass of water to call it drinkable? "Not if you're close to dying from dehydration," say some of the ranch hands. After all, the feral hogs don't seem to mind!

instructed the ranch hands not to call you names or point out obvious flaws in your character or your inability to solve simple cognitive problems like which way is up.

To remain hip and politically correct, us here at PSL Ranch are also sensitive to those easily offended by certain words. Due to several universities in Michigan and California deciding that the use of he, she, him, and her are gender micro-aggressions and offensive, we will only refer to individuals from these two states as *it* to prevent hurt feelings.

Now sit back and enjoy this somewhat twisted, demented, yet educational account of thirty-nine ways Sally met her maker as well as informative safety tips for those visiting the wild lands of Central Texas!

PSL Ranch Hands

To provide our future campers with a better understanding of each incident and to emphasize PSL Ranch's commitment to safety and a quality camping experience, we've provided a brief biography of our staff and ranch hands who have witnessed incidents throughout the years. By learning a little about each of our staff members, we think you'll feel more secure and at home on the range.

Cassandra (Cassy)

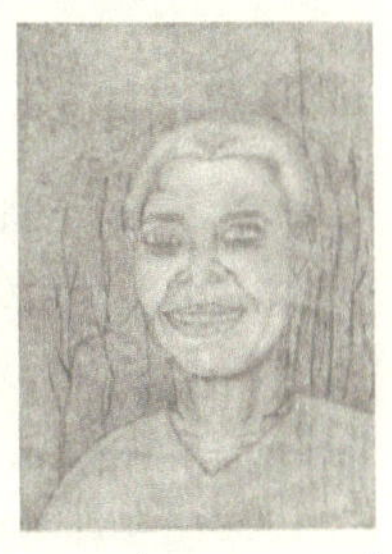

Cassy is not only PSL's camping coordinator, but a senior administrator on the ranch. Cassy hails from Jamaica, and sometimes she's hard to understand due to her heavy patois accent, particularly when she is cursing. As co-owner of the ranch, she is considered the Law of the Land, and her decisions are final (right or wrong). Cassy's favorite past times include archery, shooting at anyone she feels is a threat, and sharpening her custom-made knives.

Slim

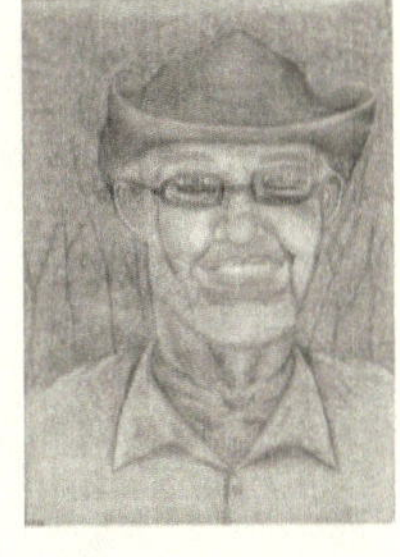

Slim is anything but slim and is also a co-owner of PSL Ranch. Slim is deathly afraid of Cassy but will assert himself when she is out of earshot. Slim is also fond of archery and shooting at anything that moves, but his main activity is killing rats and rattlesnakes when he's not fixing something on the ranch or chasing cattle away from the ranch house.

Shari Running Wild

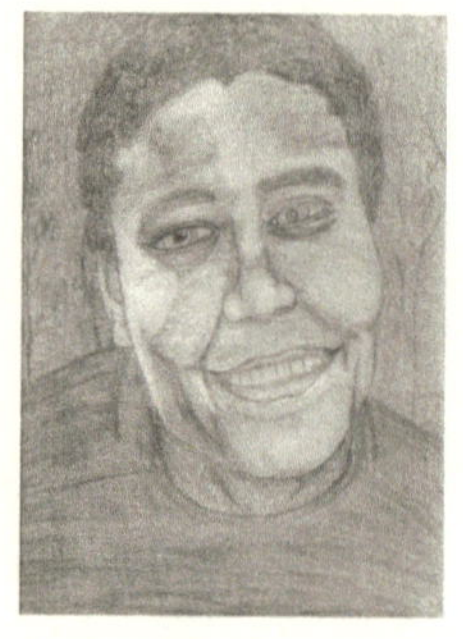

Nearly 2.4 percent Native American from an undetermined tribe, Shari Running Wild speaks in cryptic passages (no one really knows why). She is often seen hugging trees and clearing the land of rocks and dead mesquite shrubbery. Cookie and Slim have no idea who she really is or why she's even at PSL Ranch—and are afraid to ask. Shari Running Wild is an expert with a bow and a crack shot with her Chinese manufactured SKS assault rifle. The term *Injun* is no longer used at PSL Ranch as it is deemed racist and causes Shari Running Wild to shoot wildly in the direction she thinks she heard the term spoken.

Dr. S

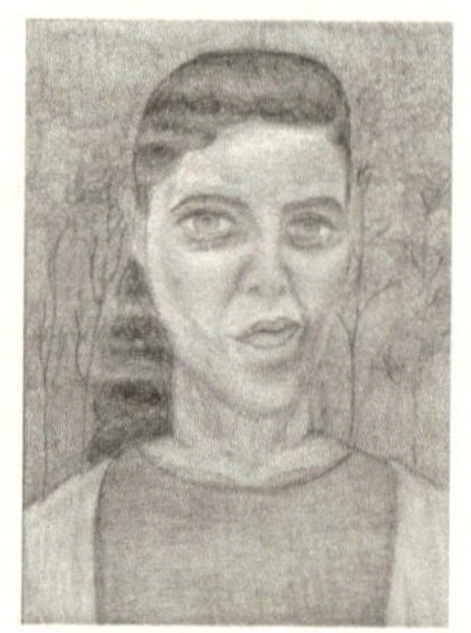

Dr. S is not someone you go to if you are sick or mortally wounded; rather, Dr. S is PSL's resident Archeologist. Although there have never been any archeological finds on PSL Ranch property, or any indication there ever will be, it only seemed appropriate to have an archeologist on staff due to the rich history of this region of the Texas Hill Country. Dr. S is an expert hog skinner and can often be spotted following Shari Running Wild around the property.

Cookie

Cookie, who is of Germanic descent, arrived at PSL Ranch to fill the role of head chef and bottle washer. Cookie rarely cooks, but when she does she spends much of her time flicking ashes from her cigars into whatever is boiling in one of her pots. After several cheap beers and a pint of schnapps, Cookie enjoys stumbling out to the campfire to relate stories of Sally's demise to visiting Junior GTCA campers. Brothers Grim would be proud of Cookie's tales as most end in death or worse!

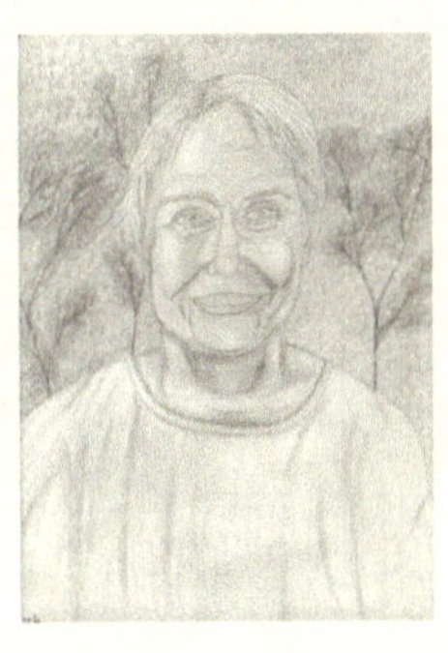

Funny Boy

Funny Boy is Dr. S's boyfriend (not sure if by choice). He hangs around Dr. S most of the time and is a comedian—literally; hence his nickname. Funny Boy's comedy skits are somewhat dark and seem to be extremely politically incorrect at times. He has often been the target of Shari Running Wild after one of his Native American jokes.

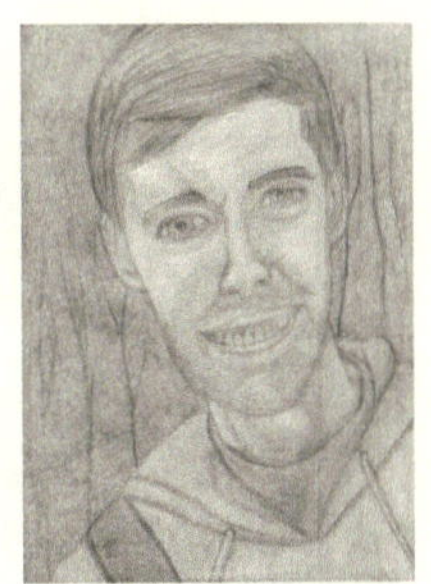

Ranch Hound (Cocoa)

PSL's ranch hound is used to track down missing campers and to ensure large predators are kept at bay. Cocoa has seventeen years of experience as PSL Ranch's hound and enjoys sleeping, not moving much, and ignoring most commands. Aside from being nearly blind, unable to smell much of anything, and deaf, his howl can be heard up to ten feet, making him a valuable asset to the team.

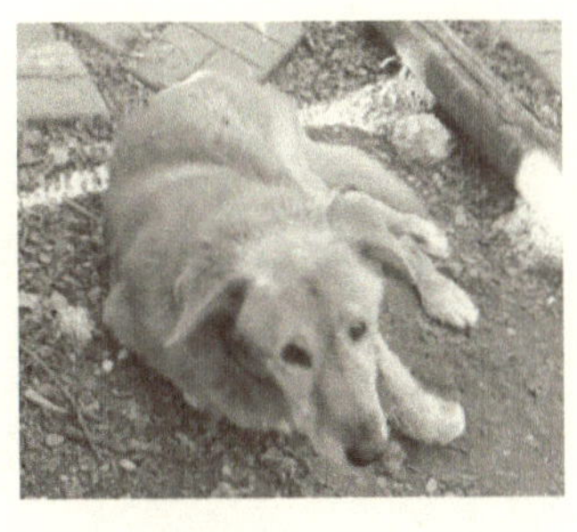

Other local characters will be mentioned from time to time such as Buck Mueller (the Menard County Sheriff), cow hands, fishermen at Cowboy Hole, or those who just stop by following an incident to see if Cassy has any of her world-famous carrot cake available for tasting (if Cookie hasn't eaten it all).

Incident #1

Death by Diamondback

GTCA Camper Receives Multiple Poisonous Snake Bites

When the owners first arrived at PSL Ranch, they spent days surveying their new acquisition. While crossing the wash and walking the fence lines, all they saw were flocks of wild turkeys, whitetail and axis deer, grey foxes, and an occasional coyote or some other predator.

At first they didn't recognize the danger, and it wasn't until some of the ranch hands began hanging dozens of diamondback rattlesnake skins from the old oak tree to dry, some six feet or more in length, that they began to be afraid—very afraid! You see, this is rattlesnake country, and they are frickin' *everywhere*!

During the first GTCA camping expedition to PSL Ranch, a group of campers took off to explore the wilds. One of the campers, Sally, didn't read the required dangerous snake pamphlet hidden in the ranch house under Cookie's booze stash. Well as bad luck would have it, Sally heard rattling from tall grass behind a brush pile. Sally, who fondly remembered the baby rattle her memaw used to put her to sleep with, ventured over with other campers to take a look. The following account of Sally's demise is described in Cookie's eyewitness account:

"I was rockin' on the cabin porch sippin' from my favorite homebrew whens I spotted through my spyglass a large diamondback coiled up and ready to strike a camper, Sally. Sally reached for a stick, but it was too late—it bit her on the arm. Worses yet, several young rattlers bit her on the leg as well. Seems she finded a nest."

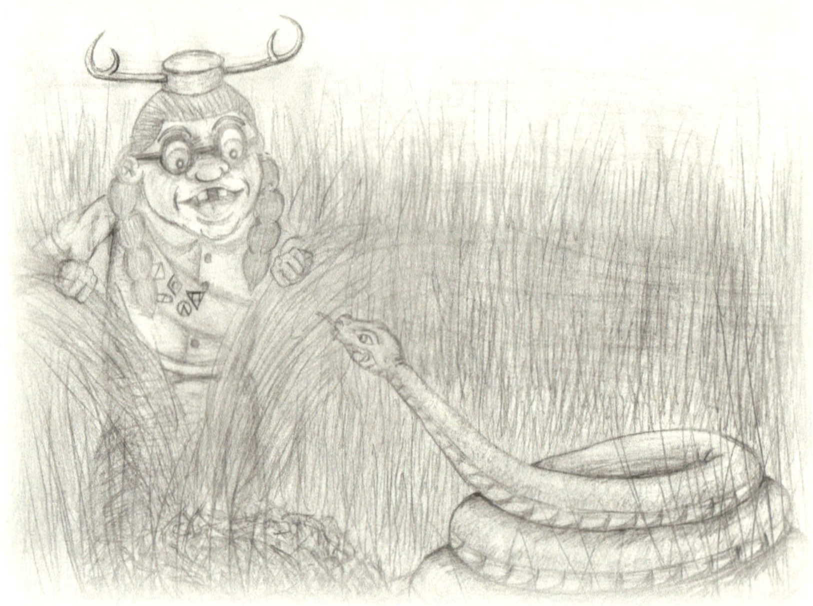

Menard County Sheriff, Buck Mueller, ruled the death accidental and PLS Ranch not liable for the following reasons:

1. The other GTCA campers seemed unaware or didn't care that Sally got bit; seems they really didn't like her anyway.
2. Cookie wasn't able to lend assistance as she had something cooking and couldn't leave the stove unattended.
3. Due to the inability to call an ambulance in a timely fashion. Sally would have died anyway.

PSL camp coordinators believe this tragic yet unavoidable death could have been prevented with a little knowledge of rattlesnakes and first aid. For instance, diamondback rattlesnakes are prolific in central Texas, and one should always be aware of his or her surroundings when walking through brush.

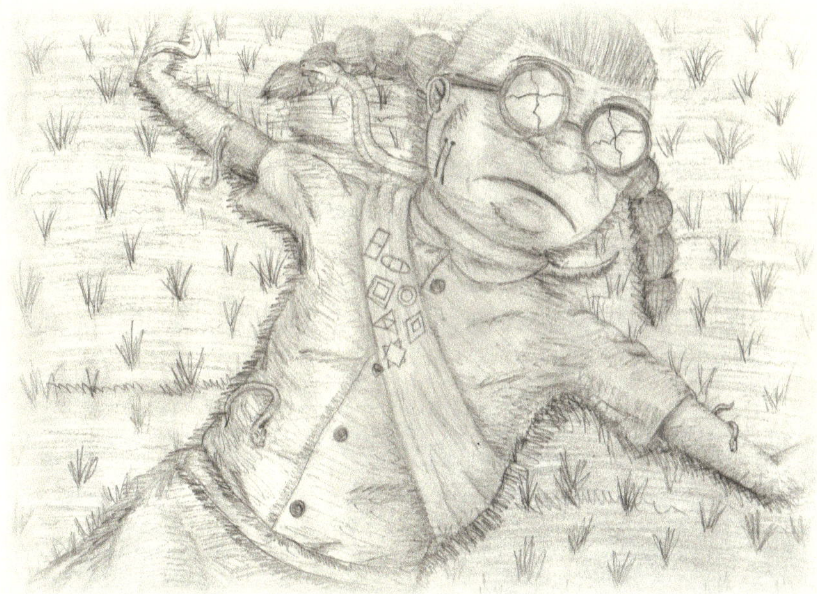

The larger diamondback rattlesnakes are not aggressive and will give you fair warning by coiling up and rattling—they don't want a fight! The smaller or baby snakes are actually more dangerous. Their rattles are quiet and difficult to hear. Furthermore, they have not learned how to control the amount of venom to release from their fangs and usually just give you a full dose!

Because you may not always be able to see or hear them, especially when Cassy and Cookie are loudly swearing at each other, proper clothing will prevent a lethal strike. Ranch hands wear knee-high snake boots that cannot be penetrated by the snake's fangs. Wearing ankle-length jeans or other leg-covering garments are also a good idea (PSL Ranch is not a good place to get a tan).

What if you do get bit? There are immediate medical procedures that can reduce the effect of the venom. First of all, most snake bites are not lethal, but you shouldn't go marching around PSL Ranch without a snake-bite kit containing a venom suction cup (we're not sucking it out for you). Also, if you witness a snake bite, it's best you lend assistance as soon as possible unless of course you have dinner on the stove.

Conclusion: Wear snake boots, stay alert, and don't approach the snakes!!

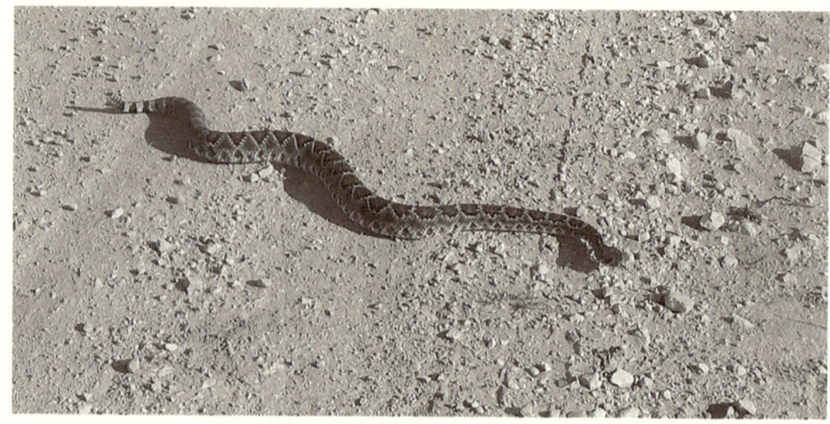

One of PSL Ranch's slithering diamondback pets

Mountain Lion Lunch

Mauling and consumption of a GTCA camper

Menard County has the dubious distinction of being one of the Texas counties that has recorded a death by mountain lion or cougar. We can only assume those counties that have not had a mountain lion incident have no one named Sally living there.

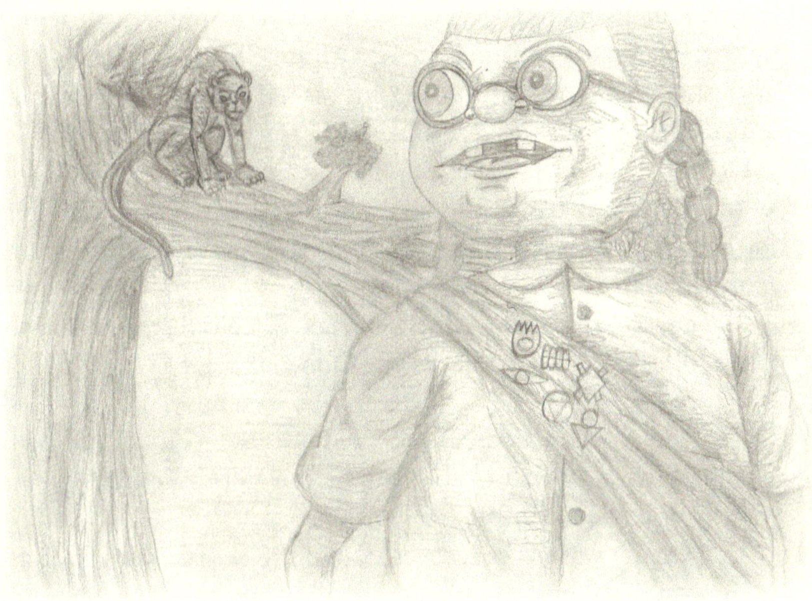

Mountain lions are stealthy hunters and attack from a tree or other high-vantage points, and usually from behind. A male can weigh up to three hundred pounds, but a female can be more lethal, especially if she is hunting or protecting her young. During an early spring campout, an unusually small Sally was hiking alone in a remote PSL ranch location where a lot of game considered tasty to mountain lions congregate. The following account of Sally's demise is described in Cassy's official eyewitness account:

"Mi a walk towaad di girl chile, wen a big puss jump outta di treetop an drop pon di likkle daalin! Mi go fi mi amma to lick im in im edback, but by di time mi tun roun di puss did eat almos aal ah di pickny and tek di res away!

English Translation: I was walking towards Sally when the cougar jumped on her. I went for my hammer to hit it in the back of the head, but when I turned around, it had eaten most of her and took the rest away.

PSL Ranch's hound, Cocoa, was called to action in an attempt to track the large cat and find the remains of Sally. After being provided Sally's scent and not moving for several hours, a search team was organized but was unsuccessful.

Dr. S was called in to accomplish an excavation of the site in order to recover any remains. She did find multiple bones and identified them as what was left of Sally, but they were later identified as old possum bones.

Menard County Sheriff, Buck Mueller, ruled the death unavoidable and PLS Ranch not liable for the following reasons:

1. Sally had wondered away from other GTCA campers, which is strictly forbidden in the GTCA camping rule book (rule #1,554).
2. A body was never recovered, and the actual cause of death could not be determined.
3. The mountain lion was hungry.

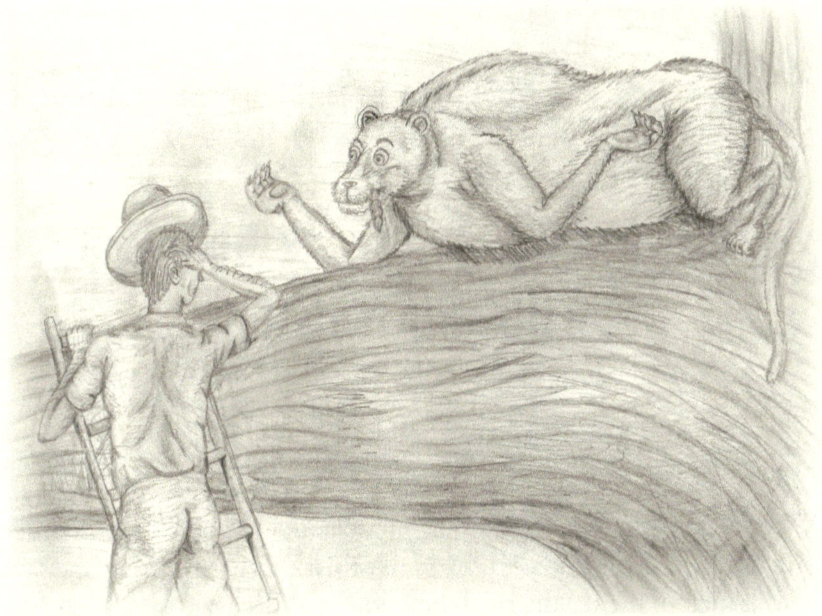

This horrific yet unavoidable incident could have been prevented with a little common sense. First of all, unless you're very familiar with the property, very attentive to your surroundings, and carry a weapon of your choice, you should not be tramping around in remote areas of PSL Ranch alone! You see, predators are less likely to eat you if you travel in groups of two or more—especially if you're small (bite-size so to speak).

To prevent similar incidents on PSL Ranch, no one is allowed to walkabout alone and must be accompanied by another camper or ranch hand (not Cookie, she'll just watch and laugh). Furthermore, before taking a hike, let someone at the ranch house know when you leave and when you expect to be back. There are also push-to-talk radios with a fifteen-mile range available to call for help if required.

Conclusion: Stay alert, hike with others, take a radio, and don't pet the cougars!

Milkweed Is Not to Be Mistaken with Milk Thistle!

Accidental consumption of Milkweed by a GTCA camper

When Cookie makes her famous potato soup, the ranch hands order out. You see, Cookie likes to add milk thistle to her recipe as she says it adds kick to the flavor. Truth be told, Cookie's liver isn't the healthiest due to a bad batch of moonshine she made, but being stubborn, she drank it all anyway. Milk thistle contains Silymarin, which is an anti-inflammatory and antioxidant. Many claim it aids people with alcohol-related liver disease, and on PSL Ranch, that means Cookie.

During a rather boring afternoon on a hot summer day, Cookie announced she was making her famous potato soup and needed a bucket of milk thistle. Well, collecting milk thistle is Funny Boy's job, but he was recently wounded by Shari Running Wild after telling a joke to Slim which included a character called "Injun Joe." You guessed it! Shari Running Wild let go with a full clip of 7.62×39 rounds from across Dry Creek where she was hugging a tree. Old Slim jumped behind the barn in time, but Funny Boy took one in his foot, and he wasn't in any mood to collect milk thistle.

The following account of what happened next is from the official investigation provided by Dr. S.

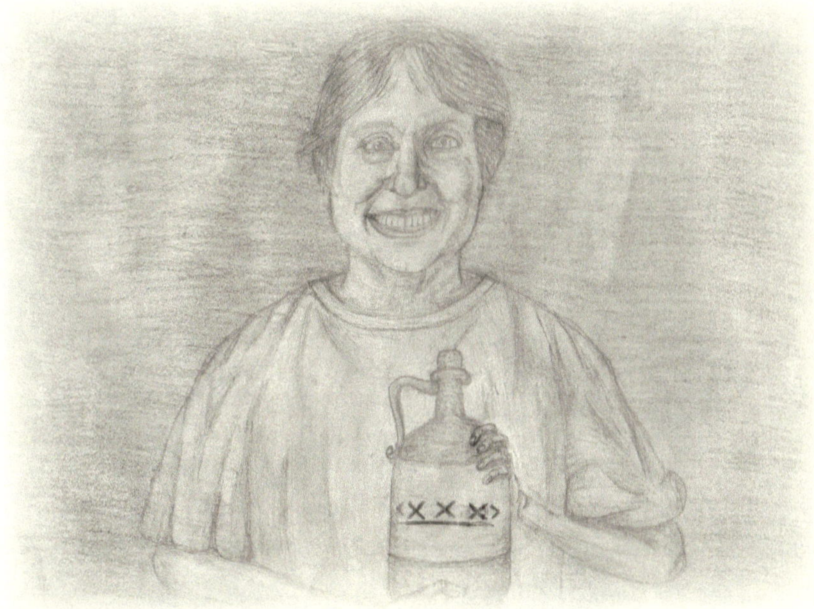

"As Funny Boy couldn't walk without crying, he hollered at nearby GTCA campers for help in collecting milk thistle. Only one, Sally, responded to his request, and she gleefully ran to him. He handed her a bucket and briefly explained between sobs what milk thistle looked like. Well, Sally went out and gathered a bucket full as fast as she could and returned to Funny Boy with her bounty. Funny Boy was in no mood to check her work as he spotted Shari Running Wild in a tree with her bow aiming at him, so he quickly said, "Take it to Cookie," and locked himself in the pump house. Cookie had just finished a pint of something strong and told Sally to *toss what she had in the pot* without first inspecting it, and Sally did. Next thing I know, Cookie passed out and Sally began sampling the soup. That evening, she howled like a coyote and kicked the bucket. It wasn't until later we found out Sally had collected milkweed, not milk thistle!"

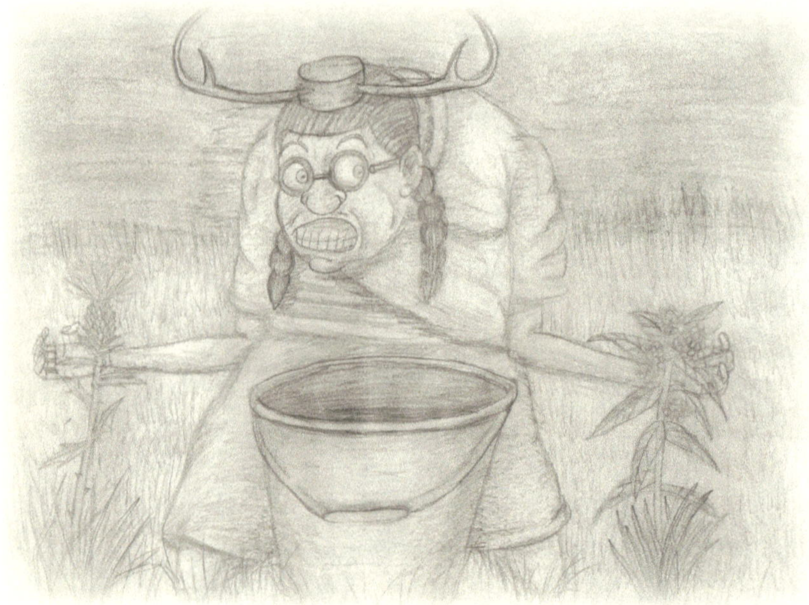

Menard County Sheriff Buck Mueller ruled the death an unfortunate act of God, and PLS Ranch was not liable for the following reasons:

1. Everyone in Menard County knows not to eat Cookie's potato soup.
2. Sally obviously flunked botany and was too ashamed to tell anyone.
3. If it's anyone's fault its Funny Boy's—he should have never told that Injun joke.

In retrospect, PSL Ranch has started educating campers on the differences between milkweed and milk thistle. While milk thistle has some unsubstantiated benefits, milkweed is in the genus Asclepias and contains cardiac glycosides, which are poisonous when eaten in large quantities.

Milkweed's toxicity depends on its species, age, and how much is consumed. Had Sally not been a pig and eaten most of the soup herself, everyone would have just gotten sick and Sally would not have expired.

Conclusion: Know what you're eating and don't eat Cookie's potato soup!

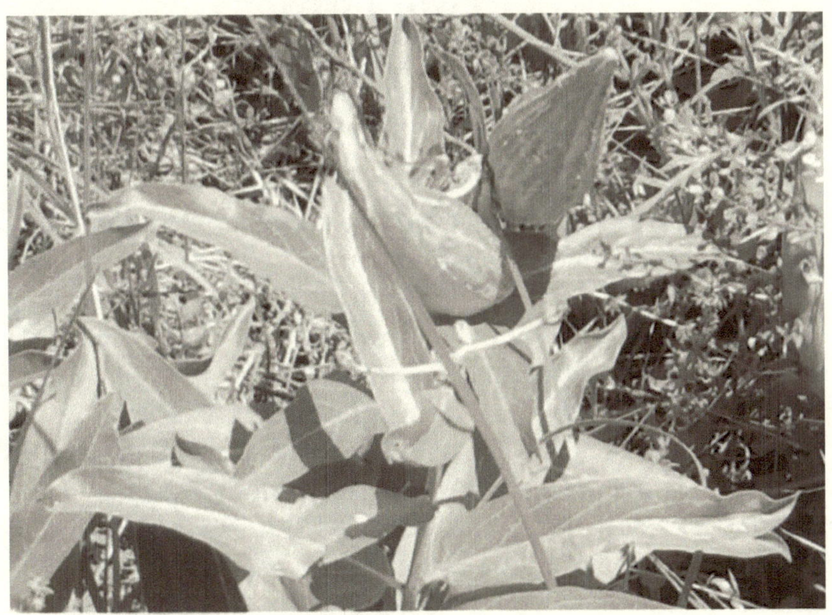

Milkweed on PSL Ranch

Incident #4

Coyote Ugly

Fatal Coyote attack on a GTCA camper

If there's one critter aside from rats, raccoons, whitetail deer, possums, and axis deer that's more prolific on PSL Ranch than rattlesnakes, it's the coyote. Coyotes are shy animals that try to avoid humans at all costs. But when their food and water is scarce, they have been known to become aggressive attacking larger prey.

During an early fall camping trip by a GTCA troop from Chicago, several campers decided to take a late afternoon stroll to the Northern edge of the ranch. Most followed the rules and stayed in groups of three or more, but one named Sally broke away to investigate a pile of brush next to an old hollow tree. There were several vultures feasting on a recently killed jack rabbit, and Sally went to chase them away.

What happened next was witnessed by Slim who provided the following statement to the Menard County sheriff's department:

"Cassy and Cookie were yelling at each other again, and Funny Boy just told another Injun joke, so the bullets were flying. I figured it was a good time to hold up a while at the bottom of the wash until all the commotion died down. It was there I saw the whole incident play out. Four, maybe ten coyotes were returning to their kill site when they spotted poor Sally. She, being a Northerner, thought all of them to be cute doggies that wanted to be petted. It all went South from there and the last thing I saw was one of them coyotes running away with a GTCA hat in its mouth. I woulda moved faster, but I could still hear hollerin' from the ranch house, so I just cowered a little while longer until I knew it was safe."

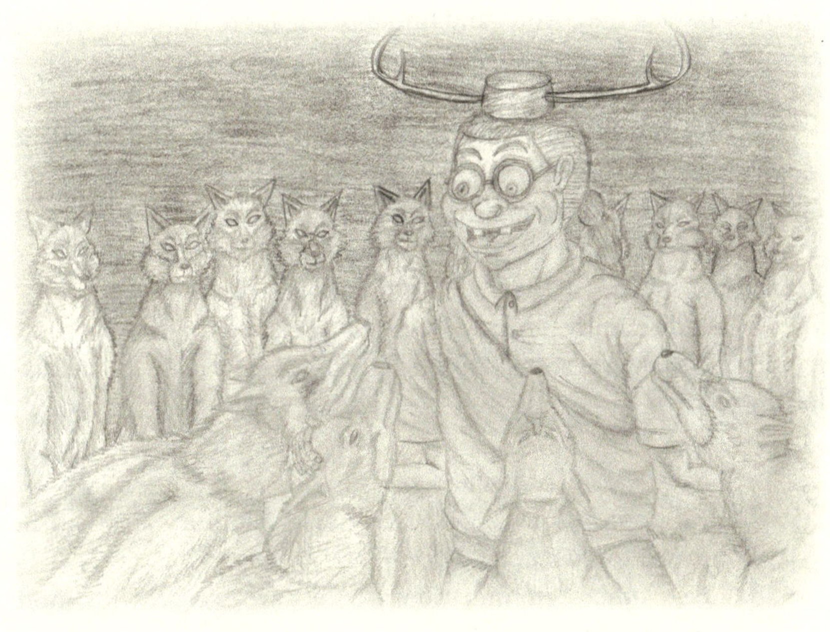

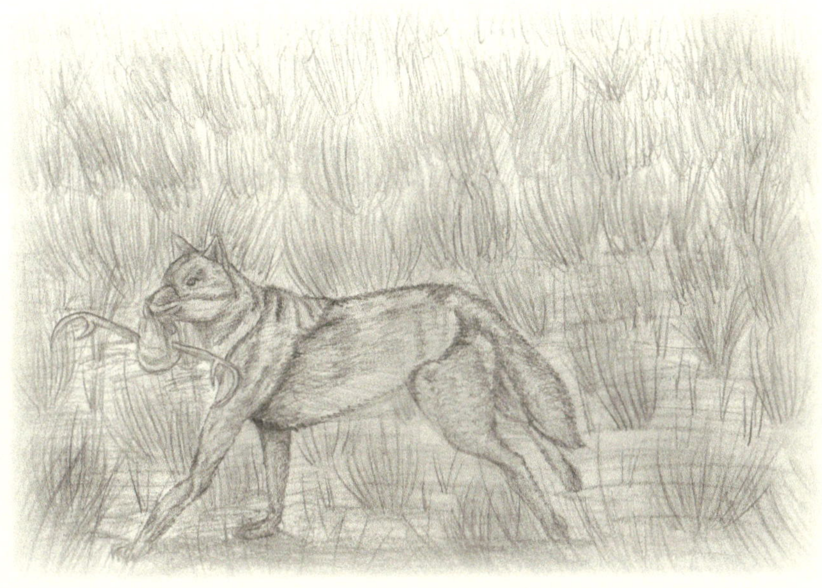

The PSL Ranch hound, Cocoa, was called to action in an attempt to track the coyotes and find the remains of Sally. After being provided Sally's scent, and not moving for several hours, a search team was organized but was unsuccessful.

Dr. S was called in by the coroner to excavate the site in order to recover any pieces of Sally that may have been left behind. After hours of work, Dr. S identified multiple bones and flesh she concluded were from Sally. It was later discovered they belonged to the dead rabbit; the coroner stated, "It was the bunny fur that indicated so."

Menard County Sheriff, Buck Mueller, ruled the incident a missing person case, and that PLS Ranch was not liable for the following reasons:

1. Sally was still missing.
2. All appropriate actions were taken by Slim, after all, he feared for his life.
3. Any other determination would have meant a lot more paperwork.

Although it was evident that PSL Ranch was not at fault, we have collected a few facts about coyotes we now pass on to our visitors:

- Coyotes generally avoid humans.
- Coyotes are wild animals and should be considered dangerous, especially if you're small!
- Never run away from a coyote—they will consider you prey.
- Making noise usually keeps them at a distance.
- Don't approach them if they have young or are eating.
- There have only been two recorded fatalities in North America due to coyotes—it is unknown if the victim's names were Sally.

Conclusion: *Don't pet the coyotes!*

Ancient Oaks: A Not-So-Subtle Squish

Live Oak, Dead GTCA Camper

Live oak trees grow naturally in the central Texas county of Menard, and PSL Ranch is blessed to have some of the biggest! These old giants line both sides of the wash, and no doubt their roots go deep to find scarce water. Many of these old oaks witnessed a time before white settlers; when thousands of buffalos would pass by on their way to the San Saba River, just four miles away, followed by Native Americans in search of a meal. Of course, these huge ancient oaks have very large limbs that measure forty to eighty inches around, and some of the lower branches are dead. For this reason, Shari Running Wild takes extreme caution when hugging one of them.

On one fateful GTCA camping expedition on PSL Ranch, a young camper named Sally decided to get some shade under one of our more ancient oaks. It was a rather windy afternoon, and the trees could be seen swaying a little more than usual. As Sally tried to smush butterflies with a stick, she failed to hear the crackling sound of a large branch thirty feet directly above her. The following eyewitness account of what happened next is provided by PSL ranch hand, Funny Boy:

"I was practicing my latest skit about Inju—… I mean, Native Americans, when I heard a cracking sound just South of the ranch house. I looked over just as a large limb from the oldest oak on the Ranch broke off in a sudden gust of wind and squished poor little Sally! All I saw were two legs and two arms stretched out on both sides covered with butterflies. I immediately thought, "What a skit this will make!"

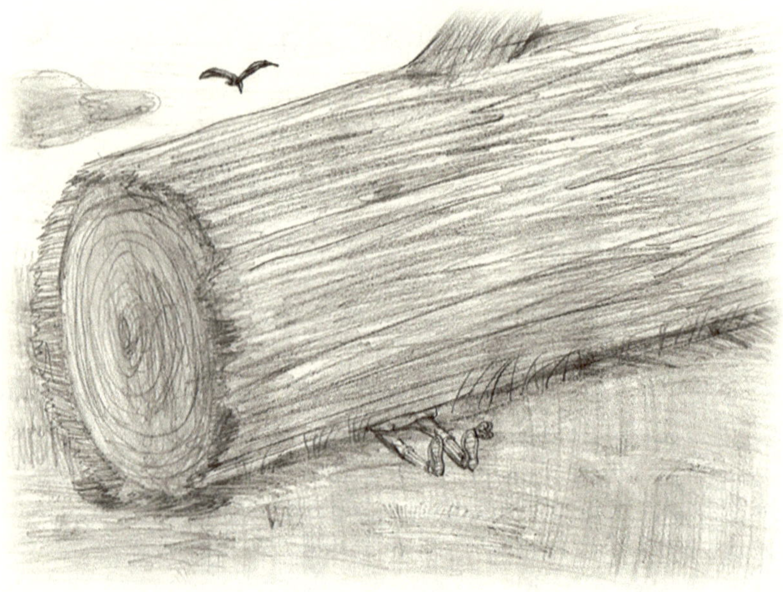

Menard County Sheriff, Buck Mueller, ruled the incident an unfortunate bizarre accident and that PLS Ranch was not liable for the following reasons:

1. Sally shouldn't have been swatting butterflies—that's just not right!
2. Sally should have been more attentive and noticed all the other limbs lying around her.
3. These things happen.

It is reported that there are over 250 billion trees in America today; in fact, there are more trees in America today than there were over one hundred years ago. Nearly one hundred people are killed by falling trees and limbs annually, and caution should be taken when moving under untrimmed trees just to be safe. Prior to this incident, Slim had seen the movie *Lord of the Rings* and now sleeps with a chainsaw in case the trees start to move toward the cabin. Slim often has nightmares and can be heard muttering, "the Ents are coming," in his sleep.

Conclusion: Be aware of your surroundings and don't smush the butterflies!

INCIDENT #6

A Stuffed Raccoon is a Safe Raccoon

Rabid raccoon, zombie camper

Raccoons are numerous on PSL Ranch and can be quite an annoyance as they tend to get into just about everything. Visitors to our ranch can spot them early in the morning or late in the evening usually around the trash bin or eating free corn at the deer feeder. Although some folks have made them into pets, such as President Calvin Coolidge, it is not recommended as they tend to remain in a wild state. Raccoons are also a favorite subject for a local taxidermist who displays them in rather unnatural settings; making them seem more cuddly and cute than ever.

On a recent GTCA campout on PSL Ranch, many of the hikers took a trip to the deer feeder one cool evening to watch the local wildlife as the sun set over the horizon. There were deer, squirrels, turkeys, and of course, a lot of raccoons. As the campers watched from a distance, one of the little furry critters was acting oddly, and the other raccoons were running away from it.

Believing that these little furry animals were friendly, one camper named Sally began to approach the feeder chasing all of the animals away except for the oddly acting raccoon, which began to approach the campers hissing and stumbling along the way.

All of the campers except Sally ran screaming back to their campsite, which seemed like a normal reaction, but Sally wanted to pet the little furry guy! What happened next was witnessed by Dr. S who happened to be in the area while following Shari Running Wild:

30

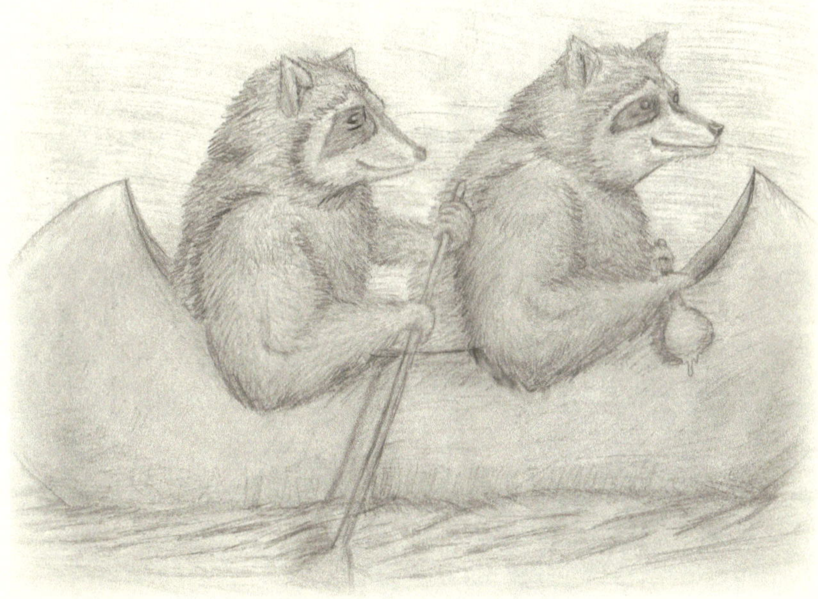

"I really couldn't see what was happening at first as the sun had just set over the horizon and the grass was tall due to recent rains. All I saw was Sally bending over to touch something, and then she jumped back and screamed! I would have followed her to see what was wrong, but then I saw Shari Running Wild performing a native dance, and I went back to observing her".

It was several weeks later when PSL Ranch administrators learned that Sally had been put down in her hometown of Saint Louis. Apparently, the local populous had just watched an episode of *The Walking Dead* when Sally was spotted on the street stumbling, hissing, and frothing at the mouth. Thinking she was a zombie, they dispatched her with an arrow to the head.

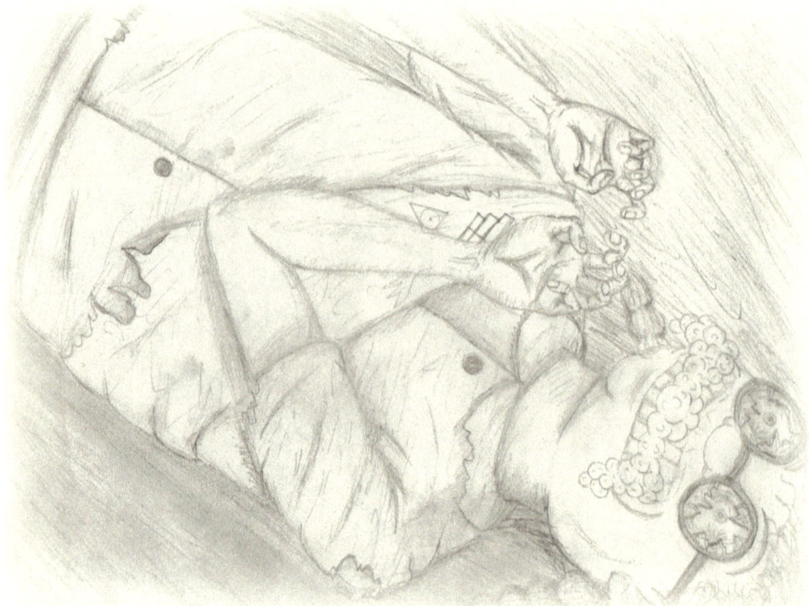

The official investigation led back to Menard County Sheriff, Buck Mueller, who ruled the incident a justifiable homicide and that PLS Ranch was not liable for the following reasons:

1. Sally wasn't killed on PSL Ranch.
2. Raccoons are for stuffing, not petting.
3. Zombies must be put out of their miseries.

In order to reduce the threat of zombie-ism on PSL Ranch, we now provide information about raccoons to our visitors. For instance, raccoons do not attack humans unless rabid. Raccoons are not aggressive or violent unless you corner them or directly threaten, or attack them. The worst injury you could suffer from a healthy raccoon are scratches, bites, or cuts.

Conclusion: Don't pet a raccoon unless it's stuffed!

Are EpiPens Really Too Expensive: Bees and Wasps
GTCA Camper Death Due to Anaphylactic Shock

Bees, wasps, and all sorts of stinging insects are numerous throughout central Texas, and PSL Ranch is no exception. These little critters don't bother anyone who doesn't bother them first! The honey bees in particular are welcome sights as they cross-pollinate all of the wild flowers that bring us such joy in the spring and early summer. Still, they can sting unannounced if you happen to walk through an area where they are particularly active.

On one summer afternoon, a bored GTCA camper, named Sally, was too lazy to join her fellow campers on a hike to the North rim of the Ranch. Instead, she moped around the ranch house until she noticed Cookie's honey supply; a rather large honey beehive about thirty feet from the cabin. Being a curious and naughty child, she pretended it was a piñata and grabbed a stick to give it a whack.

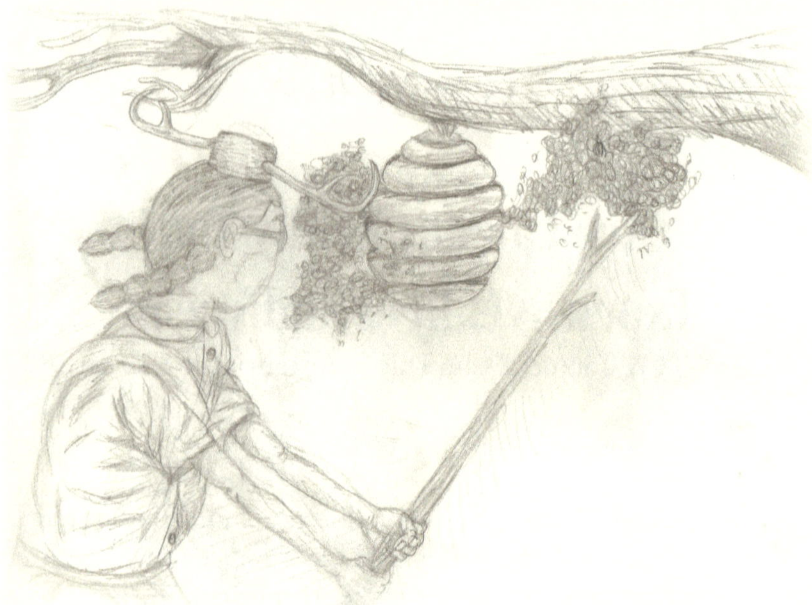

The following eye witness testimony was provided to the Menard County Sherriff's Department by Funny Boy who witnessed the fateful event:

"I was hiding under the cabin to prevent a direct shot from Shari Running Wild. When I looked up to see what all the commotion was about. I saw the camper in question swinging left and right trying to hit Cookie's beehive. I would have told her to stop, but I didn't want to give my position away, fearing for my life and all. Anyway, Sally swung and swung until she finally connected with a direct shot! The bees were already agitated by her actions, but once she clobbered the hive, they took action and stung her by the thousands! She immediately fell over and blew up like a balloon of many colors! By the time I felt safe enough to lend a hand, she was already dispatched by the angel of death. What a skit this will make!"

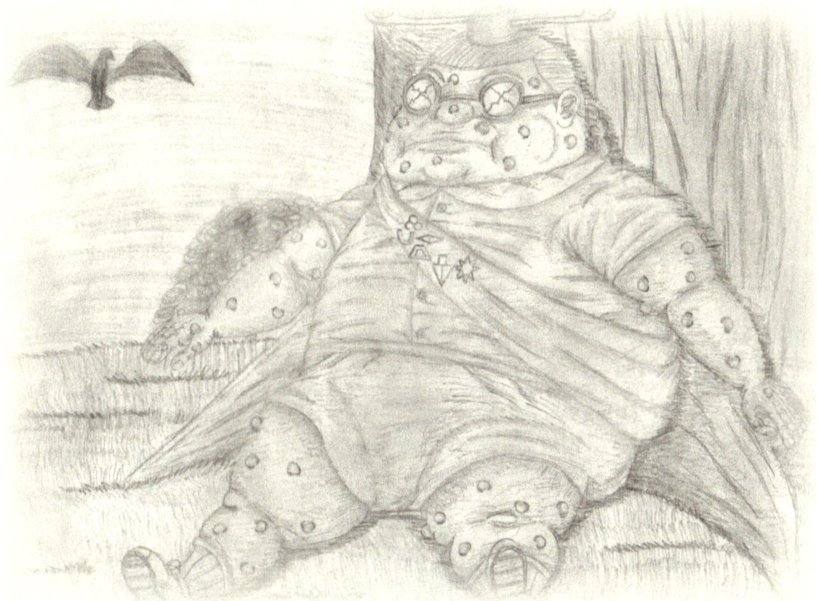

Apparently, Sally was deathly allergic to bee stings. During the investigation, it was discovered that Sally's parents didn't want to dish out $600 for an EpiPen. Sally's father was quoted as saying, "I had ten kids, and now I have nine, but I still have $600 to my name!"

Menard County Sheriff, Buck Mueller, ruled the incident a case of stupidity and that PLS Ranch was not liable for the following reasons:

1. Sally's parents weren't really that concerned but should have provided the appropriate medical device for a camping trip.
2. Funny Boy was in a predicament and could not have rendered assistance; after all, he feared for his life.
3. If Sally hadn't died from the bee stings, Cookie would have certainly killed her for destroying her source of honey.

Although PSL Ranch was cleared of any wrongdoing, we now provide some facts about bee stings for our visitors:

1. According to the Center for Disease Control, bees are the deadliest non-human animal in America.
2. Fifty people die each year from bee stings, and the number is increasing due to the aggressive Africanized honey bees that are taking over Texas.
3. Lightning kills more people than bees each year (around ninety).
4. Bee stings are not deadly unless you are allergic to them.
5. If you are allergic to bee stings, you should have the appropriate medical devices handy to prevent anaphylaxis.

We hope these facts will quell any fears you might have about visiting our beautiful Texas countryside. When visiting PSL Ranch, it's a good idea not to mention this incident to Cookie, she still gets mighty agitated about the loss of her honey source!

Conclusion: Don't swat the bees!

Bobcat—Not Your Average Pussycat

Bobcat Attack on a GTCA Camper

Bobcats in central Texas are smaller than their Northern cousins; reaching a top weight of only thirty pounds. They are normally hard to find as they are stealthy, quiet, and avoid humans at all costs. They usually go after very small game, such as rats, squirrels, and birds, but have been known to attack larger prey when their usual prey is scarce.

Several years ago, during a late winter GTCA expedition to PSL Ranch, a camper named Sally found a can of squirrel urine that is normally used to bait coyotes. Being adventurous and disobedient, Sally crept out of her tent past curfew in the middle of the night to spray the nasty smelling bait on one of the dead oak trees at the base of the wash, far out of sight from the other campers and PSL ranch hands. Sally, being height challenged (we don't use the term midget—it's just plain rude), hid on the far side of a large log and began spraying the squirrel urine in the wind.

What happened next was witnessed by Cassy who just happened to be down the wash a bit practicing some voodoo ritual, which consisted of hitting a Slim doll with a stick while chanting, "The Ents are coming."

"Mi si di puss dem crouch low pon de gras staakin dem pray. Mi tink a wat dat pus up to, so mi watch it. When all of a sudden di puss drop down pon sumting an mi hear di poor pickny holla an run like di devil hot pon are trail. Mi wudda elp are but mi magic na finish by itself."

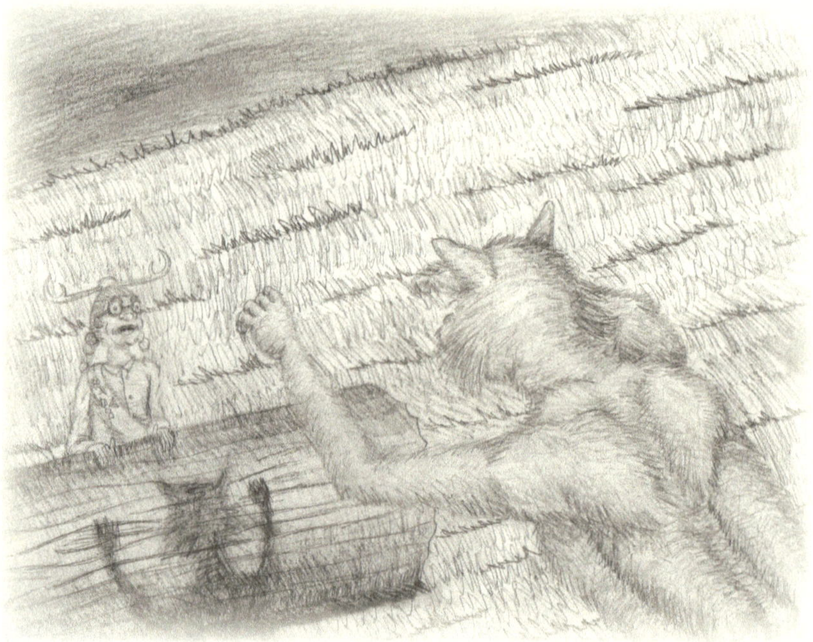

English Translation: "I saw the bobcat crouching as if to strike something, so I looked on to see what it was up to. Suddenly, it pounced on something, and I heard Sally yelp and run away. I would have followed but it was dark, and I had to finish my magic.

Apparently, the bobcat was attracted by the squirrel urine spray and thought a squirrel would make a great late-night snack. Unfortunately for Sally, it struck her femoral artery before realizing Sally wasn't a squirrel; just a height-challenged camper with a can of squirrel urine. Sally was discovered the following day at the far Southwest corner of the ranch, dead due to blood loss.

Menard County Sheriff, Buck Mueller, who was a little pissed-off because his fishing trip had been interrupted, ruled the incident another unfortunate act of nature and that PLS Ranch was not liable for the following reasons:

1. Sally broke curfew, which is a gross violation of GTCA rule #324.

2. Sally stole the can of squirrel urine from Cookie's seasoning supplies.
3. It was only natural for a bobcat to attack something that short.

Taking no responsibility for this incident, PSL Ranch administrators decided to provide some facts about bobcats for future visitors in order to alert them to possible danger. Most notably, there has never been a recorded death of a human from a bobcat attack in North America until now.

Attacks are rare and have been associated with cornering one or, you guessed it, baiting one who then thinks you're something you're not! Bobcats have attacked prey as large as a deer, but usually when the deer is sick or otherwise compromised and cannot flee. Smaller farm animals, such as baby goats (kids), are also taken as food from time to time.

Conclusion: Don't piss in the wind!

INCIDENT #9

Toadstools Are Not Mushrooms

The Death of a GTCA Hiker Due to Consumption of Toadstools

One of the educational activities on PSL Ranch is to gather local foodstuffs for a campfire meal. This includes herbs and plants that will enhance one of Cookie's bland meals while at the same time dampening the taste of her cigar ash. Each camper is provided a guide of edible plants and critters, and sent on their way.

On one such expedition to acquire tasty morsels, a GTCA camper named Sally happened onto a batch of what she thought to be mushrooms. Sally always ordered double mushrooms on her pizza, so she picked every one she could find and rushed back to camp to prepare her prize. Once Cookie served up her mystery goulash, Sally threw in her "mushrooms" and began eating furiously.

What happened next was witnessed by Slim, who was enjoying his store-bought food by the campfire with Sally and other GTCA campers:

"Most of the PSL Ranch hands use hot sauce by the jar-full to kill the taste of Cookie's cookin' while most of the campers just throw their food in the fire and eat junk food sent by their folks back home, but Sally et the meal like there was no tomorrow! After about thirty minutes, she begin a groanin' and fartin' up a storm. The campfire was a blazin', and when Sally tried to get up, she turned her back to the fire and what came out of that little gal's rear-end was sumthin' terrible! Next thin' I know, her gas caught fire and Sally blew up! There were pieces of that little girl all over the place!"

40

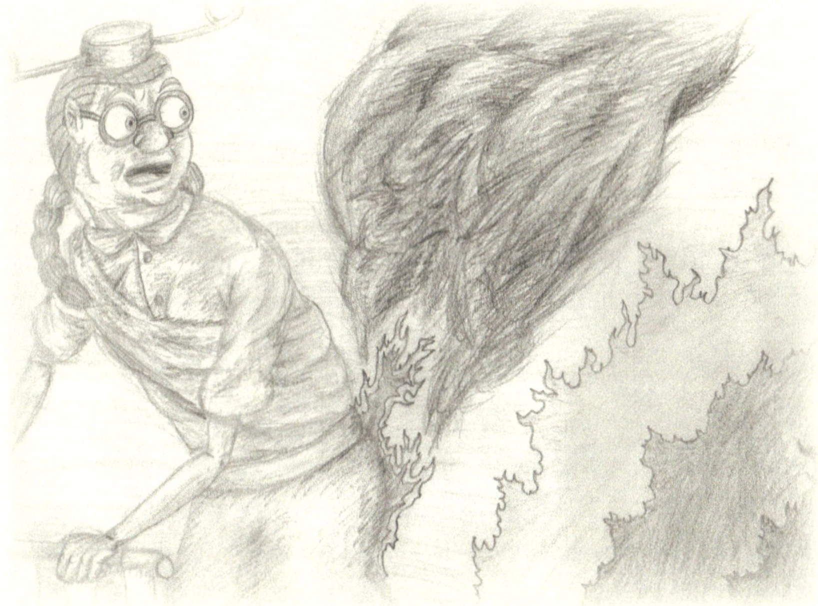

Sally was no more, but enough remains were recovered by the ranch hound allowing for an investigation. Some of the remains indicated the culprit: toadstools.

Menard County Sheriff, Buck Mueller, ruled the incident a case of poor choice, and that PLS Ranch was not liable for the following reasons:

1. Sally's parents didn't send her junk food, thereby putting her at risk of Cookie's cooking.
2. Sally should have asked a ranch hand if what she collected was edible.
3. It couldn't be determined if the intense methane cloud emanating from Sally's behind was actually caused by the toadstools in question.

Although Sheriff Mueller's points were all valid, and it was definitely not PSL Ranch's fault Sally exploded, camp coordinators nonetheless felt they should further educate future campers of the difference between mushrooms and toadstools as well as Cookie's meals and edible food.

After careful review of the scientific evidence, there is really no difference between a mushroom and a toadstool as looks can be deceiving unless you are an expert. The terms are often interchangeable as they refer to the same types of fungus. In common talk, the term toadstool usually refers to the poisonous types of fungus, and the term mushroom is used for the edible fungus.

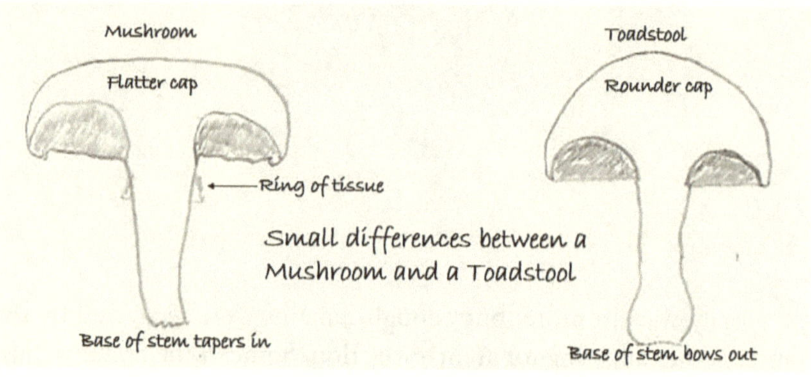

Some names for toadstools such as Devil's droppings, are usually indicators of the poisonous varieties and should be avoided. If you eat the poisonous variety of fungus, symptoms range from a mild upset stomach to severe gastrointestinal distress like Sally had. Other issues that can arise include:

- Internal hemorrhage
- Kidney or liver failure
- Confusion and anxiety

Other pleasant-looking morsels should be avoided as well. There are a variety of bushes and plants that have beautiful little red berries that look as if they belong on your morning cereal, but in fact, they will kill you! One such plant that grows in abundance on PLS Ranch is called Texas Nightshade (Solanum spp.), and only a handful of these berries can cause death! Symptoms can be immediate or take hours after munching the little buggers. So if you think you ate some, get a checkup before the symptoms begin!

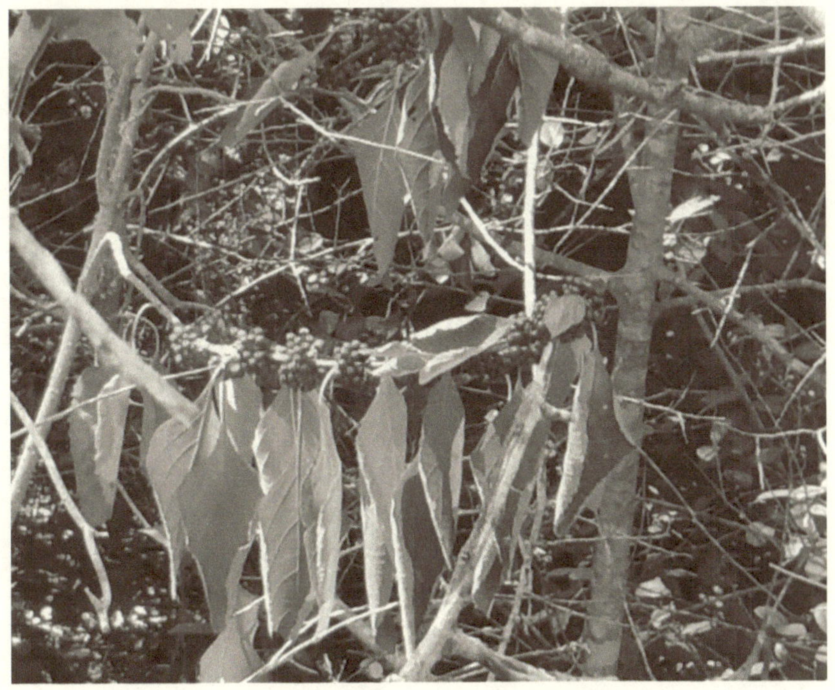

Texas Nightshade on PSL Ranch

Conclusion: Season Cookie's meals with hot sauce!

Incident #10

Signal Up High

The Falling Death of a GTCA Camper

The beautiful old live oaks of central Texas stretch and linger as they extend their large limbs to great distances, providing wide-wooden walkways for the daring. Many of the old majestic trees on PSL Ranch consist of two or more trunks veering off in opposite directions, allowing Shari Running Wild to easily climb the trunks to the higher limbs; which provided her an excellent view of the land that was once her forefathers'; well, at least 2.4 percent of her forefathers.

Although Shari Running Wild makes climbing the old live oaks look easy, it still takes practice, and she must be attentive to each foothold lest she fall. Other distractions are found in trees to include squirrels, bird nests, and of course, the bull snakes that climb the trees to eat the squirrel's young and the bird's eggs. There are also rascally raccoons hiding in the crevices during the day waiting for their chance to raid the camper's food stores each night.

One summer eve, a GTCA college student from Michigan, named Sally, who volunteered as a GTCA chaperone was irritated that there was no cellular service to be found on PSL Ranch and decided to rectify the situation by climbing the tallest live oak. Sally was what you might consider an activist and was having a less than enjoyable time with all of the local Texans who used so many micro aggressions in their everyday conversations. Yes, ma'am; no, sir, and

44

other cruel and insensitive terms are commonly used in Texas, and to it[2], it was intolerable!

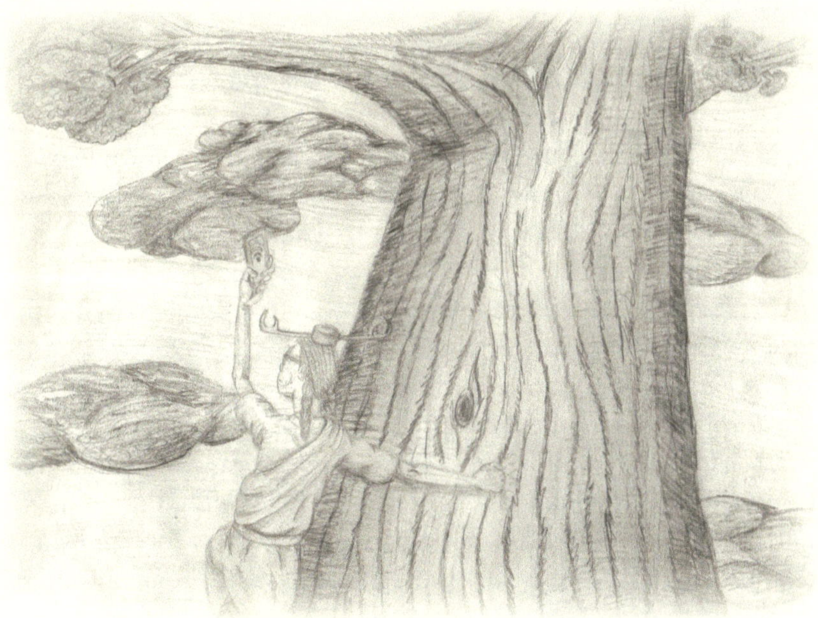

With its cell phone in hand, it climbed and climbed until it had reached the highest limb a Northern city it could reach. What happened next was witnessed by Shari Running Wild who was sitting thirty feet above it when the incident occurred. Shari Running Wild's lengthy meticulous account was provided to the Menard County sheriff's department:

"It climb, it fall, it dead."

Apparently, it was not the climber it thought it was and fell over thirty feet to it's death. It was never understood if it was spooked by a critter or just lost it's balance, but the result was one less it on PSL Ranch.

[2.] To fully understand our use of the gender-neutral term 'it', please refer to the Introduction.

Menard County Sheriff, Buck Mueller, ruled the incident a case of improper balance, and that PLS Ranch was not liable for the following reasons:

1. It should have been tending to the younger GTCA campers and not checking tweets.
2. It was a college student and it should have known better.
3. There is no entry for *it* in the official *Texas Accidental Death* paperwork, therefore, no entry could be made.

We at PSL Ranch feel awful about what happened to it, but this is proof that even those portending to be adults can come to a quick end when they are not careful climbing the old live oaks. To decrease the possibility of another politically correct death on PSL Ranch, the ranch hands have built steps on several of the easier to climb trees to provide a safer alternative to free climbing. It should be further noted that it never did find the signal it was looking for—at least in this life! Here are some rather enlightening facts about injury and death due to trees:

* Annually, 5,600 children die or are injured in tree related accidents.
* Falls are the second-leading cause of death from unintentional injury in the US.
* Over 36 percent of all hunting deaths in Georgia are caused by falling out of trees (it is Georgia after all).
* Tree climbing is so dangerous lumberjacks cannot get insurance.
* The professional tree climber's organization, Tree Climbers International, recommends against free climbing trees because it is so dangerous.

Conclusion: There is no cell service on PSL Ranch!

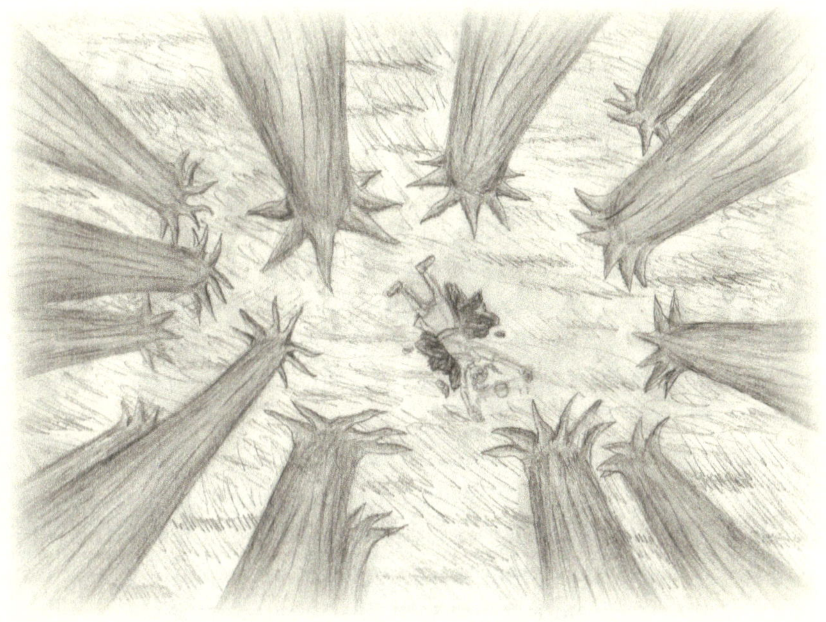

INCIDENT #11

Jumping Rocks

Death of a GTCA Hiker Due to a Rock Attack

Around 65–145 million years ago, the Cretaceous period shaped the landscape of PSL Ranch. Early on, the shoreline of the Gulf was in the South Central Texas area, but by 100 million years ago the ranch was a shallow sea and covered by thick layers of marine calcareous sediment (limestone for those of you in California). Central Texas slowly lowered over the next few million years, so the sea level rose. By the Late Cretaceous period, the sea covered almost all of Texas and extended to the North Pacific Ocean. Hundreds of feet of limestone, chalk, and mudstone accumulated over the ranch location during this time.

Glaciers never made it this far South, but there were volcanoes to the West that deposited other minerals across the landscape. As the limestone and mud deposits hardened and became brittle, continental shifts and vegetation broke up much of the surface rock into all different-sized boulders and stones. Torrential rains over millions of years also changed the landscape and created our wash (sometimes referred to as Lake Rohret).

Some of the ranch hands, particularly Cassy, believe the rocks at PSL Ranch have a mind of their own and do not appreciate human occupation. Cassy often complains about *jumping rocks* that reach out and bite her on the shin, leaving nasty bruises and the occasional laceration. On one fateful morning, such an event took place taking the life of an unsuspecting GTCA camper, named Sally, as she strayed from an approved hiking trail. The following eyewitness testimonial was provided to the Menard County sheriff's department by Cookie:

48

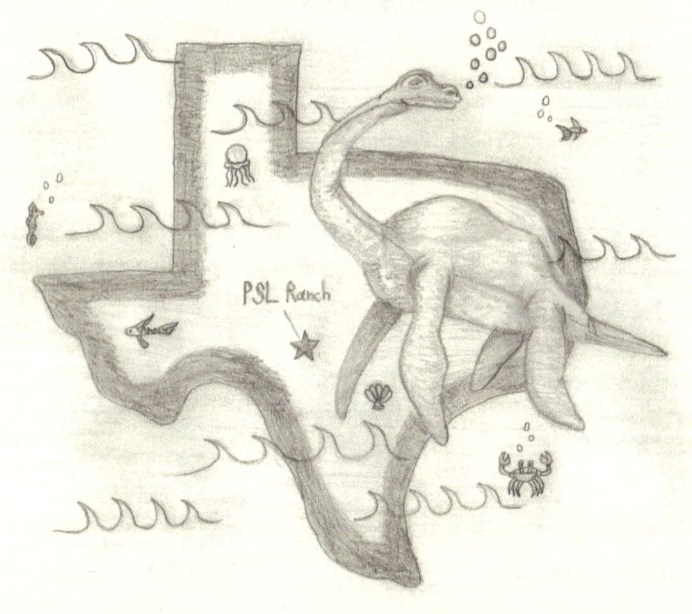

"I was out findin' a new spot fur my still as the feds recently raided my old one, and that wuddn't due no more. That's when I saws them nosey campers commin' down the trail, so I hid myself behind an old log. One of them, I thoughts it was Sally, was skippin' and jumpin' all over the place not watchin' where she was goin'. All of a sudden like, I hear her yell and start jumpin' on one leg, then she yelled again and switched up her jumpin' legs. Then she leaped, and a boulder I ain't never seen there before cracked her on her neck. The yelling stopped, so I go over nice and careful-like as there are large rocks all over the place hiding just under the grass where ya can't see um. There laid poor Sally, broke neck and all; lifeless as the rocks around her!"

After a careful examination by the Menard County Coroner's office, it was determined that Sally had died from a broken neck. She also had several severe bruises and lacerations on both legs, probably due to rocks in the vicinity.

Menard County Sheriff, Buck Mueller, ruled the incident a stone-cold case of bludgeoning, and that PLS Ranch was not liable for the following reasons:

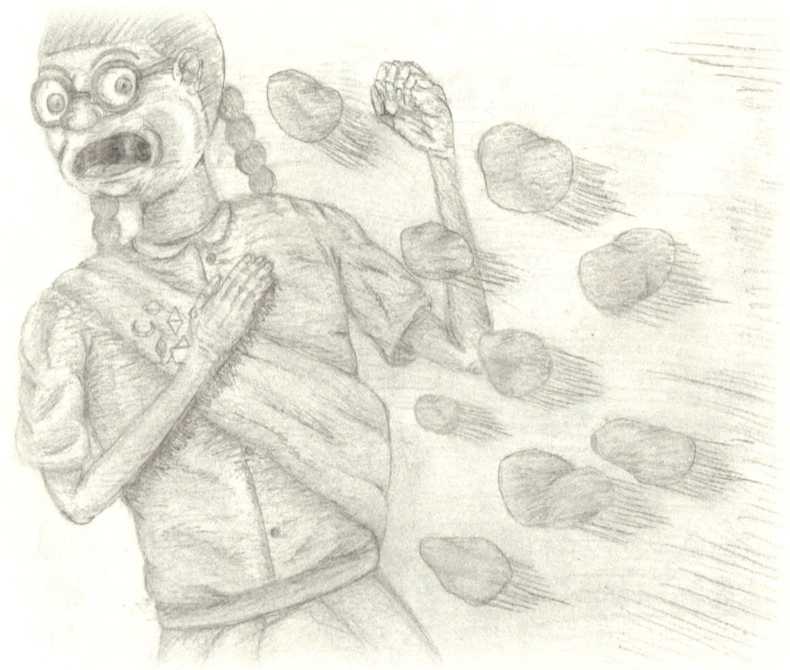

1. Sally should have stayed on the approved hiking trails.
2. PSL Ranch hand Cassy warned each camper about the jumping rocks, usually as a story around the campfire.
3. Rocks cannot be charged with murder in Menard County, but had this incident occurred in neighboring Schleicher County, that boulder would have been tried, sentenced, and crushed into gravel!

Over twenty-one Americans have died from rock incidents. Most of these were due to the victims falling onto them when they were rock climbing; still, it was never proven that the killer rocks did not move underneath them as they fell. PSL Ranch administrators feel really bad about what happened to Sally, and although PSL

Ranch takes absolutely no responsibility for this unfortunate case of death by jumping rocks, we felt we needed to take some precautions. Therefore, the approved trails have been better defined to prevent campers from mistakenly leaving them.

Conclusion: Watch where you step and listen closely to Cassy's tale of the jumping rocks!

Incident #12

12

The Wash

Death of a GTCA Camper Due to a Harsh Environment

Tens of thousands of years of rainfall eroded the soft limestone running directly down the middle of PSL Ranch, creating what is commonly referred to as a wash. The official definition of a wash is a dry creek bed or gulch that temporarily fills with water following heavy rains or drainage from flatlands.

Most washes are dry and barren, but not PSL Ranch's wash; it is filled with all sorts of cactus, thistles, mesquites, boulders, and a thick layer of grass. There is also a healthy population of poisonous snakes that make it their home unless it floods, at which time they climb the banks in large quantities.

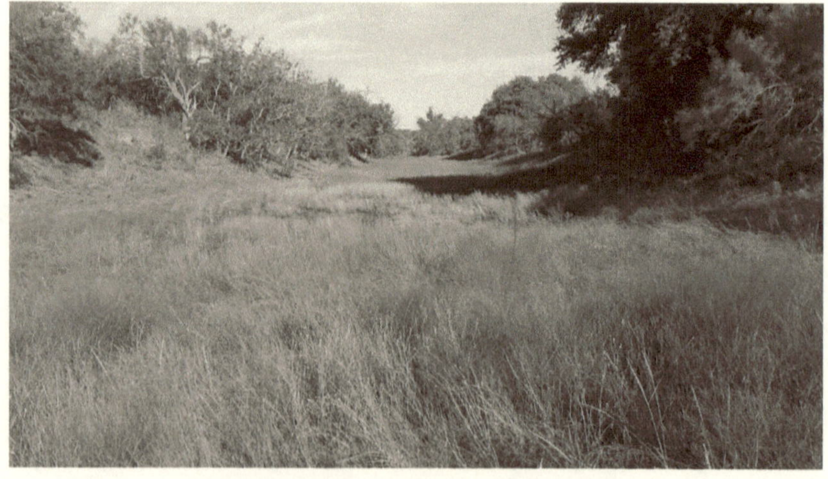

A view of PSL Ranch's Northern wash

Walking directly across PSL Ranch's wash is not advised and is rather difficult due to hidden obstacles. Furthermore, pools of water are scattered over the wash, hidden just under the grass allowing for tripping and increasing animal hazards. That's why PSL Ranch has created a trail that crosses the wash mostly unencumbered—when it's not flooded.

One late fall day around dusk, a GTCA hiking expedition was headed for the Western-most portion of PSL Ranch across the wash. The team was led by Shari Running Wild who was taking them to watch the sunset and to observe a clear sky-full of stars without the light pollution from city lights. She led the young hikers down the Western boundary of the ranch to the only approved trail that crosses the wash.

You see, not even Shari Running Wild would dare cross the wash at its closest location to the campsite as it contains too many hazards. Unfortunately, one camper named Sally decided to have three helpings of dessert, a wonderful homemade carrot cake prepared by Cassy. Cassy's carrot cake is coveted by everyone from the San Antonio River to the San Saba, and if you get a chance to have more than one piece, you take it! Unfortunately for Sally, Cassy's carrot cake was her undoing as she still intended to see the bright stars come hell or high water—she found both! What happened next was witnessed by Slim, who happened to be popping rats with his old .22 on the West bank when the incident occurred:

"I was sittin' buy an old pile of wood plinkin' rats with some rat-shot most of the evenin'. Rat-shot is fun as ya gotta be close to the little critters or it won't even hurt 'em. I sometimes use this load to shoot lazy ranch hands in the ass as it keeps them on their toes. Anyway, while I sat there, I saw somethin' small, maybe a little girl wearing one of them GCTA hats that look so stupid run out of the dining area directly down the bank of the wash into the weeds. I yelled fer her to stop, but she didn't respond! I ran over and looked down, but it was all dark and scary, so I went inside to get whatever was left of Cassy's carrot cake and some of Cookie's homebrew."

The next morning, after a good hearty breakfast of possum brains and eggs, GTCA camp counselors took role and discovered

Sally was missing! Immediately, the ranch hound was provided Sally's scent so he could hunt her down. After three to four hours of inactivity by Cocoa, a search party was led by Funny Boy to find Sally.

Sally was found face down in about a foot of water with multiple snake bites, contusions from jumping rocks, and pierced head to toe from hundreds of cactus thorns. The Menard County Coroner's office listed the official cause of death as fright.

Menard County Sheriff, Buck Mueller, ruled the incident a frightful case of bad judgement and procrastination, and that PSL Ranch was not liable for the following reasons:

1. Sally should have remained behind as she knew the expedition had left sometime earlier.
2. Everybody knows you don't cross the middle of PSL Ranch's wash, especially when it's getting dark.
3. After three pieces of Cassy's delightful carrot cake, she must have died happy!

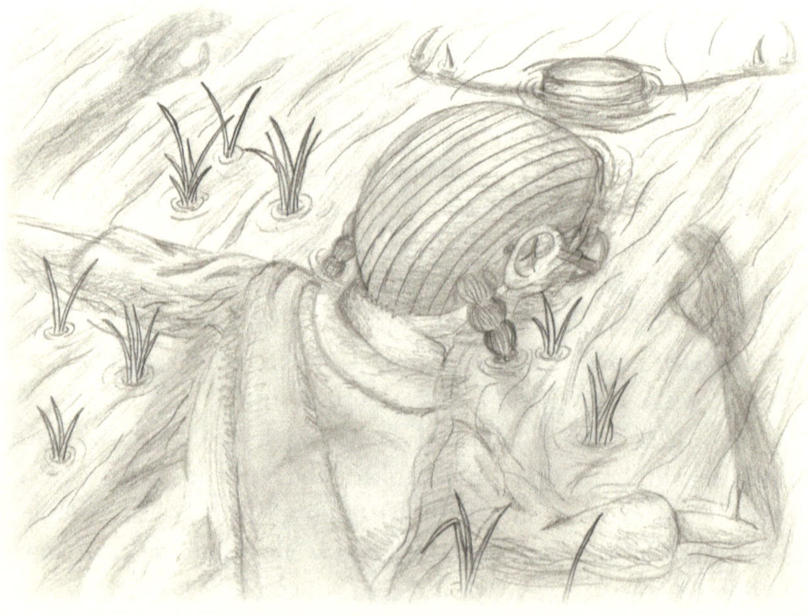

PSL Ranch administrators once again feel mighty bad about Sally's fatal attempt to meet up with the other campers, and even though it clearly was not any fault of the ranch hands, a few more facts about our wash may help to deter campers from crossing anywhere but the approved trail when they are late for an appointment.

Much of the year, the wash has water in low-lying areas, making it rather dangerous to cross for those not familiar with its features. Even ranch hands who know their way around the wash will usually avoid it as there are too many obstacles and critters that can jump out and grab you. Such obstacles include:

- Rocks and boulders that trip you or knock you in the head
- Cactus and thistles
- Logs and thick weeds that trip you
- Pools of water, from a few inches to a foot or more in depth
- Diamond back, cotton mouth, timber rattlers, and even coral snakes make the wash their home (remember, if its black and yellow it will kill a fellow)
  All sorts of critters that are looking for water, from axis deer to feral hogs

Most of these obstacles are hidden or very quiet, making it difficult for anyone to cross unhindered. It should be noted that even the approved trail can be hazardous. Snakes like basking in the sun, and because the approved path is clear of vegetation, they sometimes occupy a portion of the trail. You can easily avoid being bitten by turning around and running away (rattlers usually don't pursue)!

Conclusion: Use the approved path!

Hell, It's a Hailstorm!

Death of a GTCA Camper Due to a 60,000-Foot Cumulus Nimbus

Texas thunderstorms are legendary, and those arriving from the Western flatlands are some of the fiercest. Although it is dry most of the year in Menard County, when it rains, it pours! Even worse, tornadoes, high winds, and hail are common and should be respected. In fact, if you look closely at the local vehicles, you will often spot deep dents from hail that pockmark the vehicle from an earlier storm.

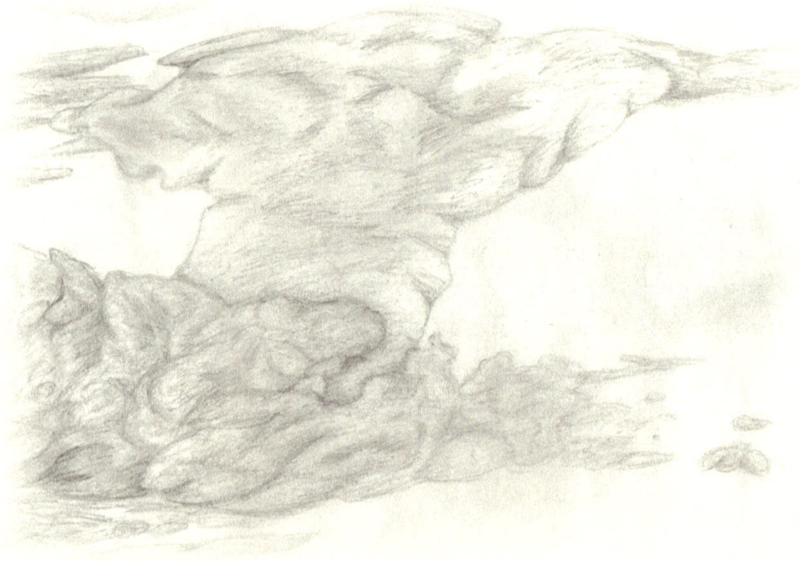

What makes the hail in Central and South Texas so large and solid is the immense size of the storms in which they are formed. The farther South you go, the taller the Cumulus Nimbus. They have been recorded as high as 75,000 feet in the tropics and are usually between 40–60,000 feet in Central Texas (for the bigger storms). When conditions are right and a big storm emerges, hail stones the size of your fist can develop as they are tossed up and down in the massive clouds, freezing and growing until they are released on the unsuspecting below.

One such storm formed not long ago and PSL Ranch was in its crosshairs! This was a particularly bad storm as the hailstones were irregular due to that fact that multiple stones froze together to form an oblong shape with sharp edges; commonly referred to as devil stones. It was a beautiful storm that could be viewed end to end with a large anvil reaching over 40,000 feet in the sky. Slim saw the orange tint in the upper third of the anvil and immediately knew he needed to send out the alarm as this storm contained hail!

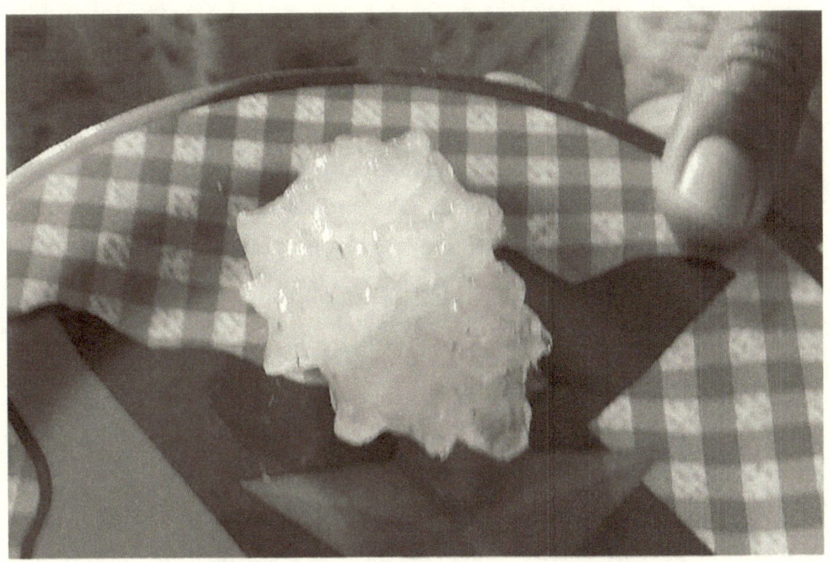

Actual Devils Stone held by PSL Ranch hand Cassy

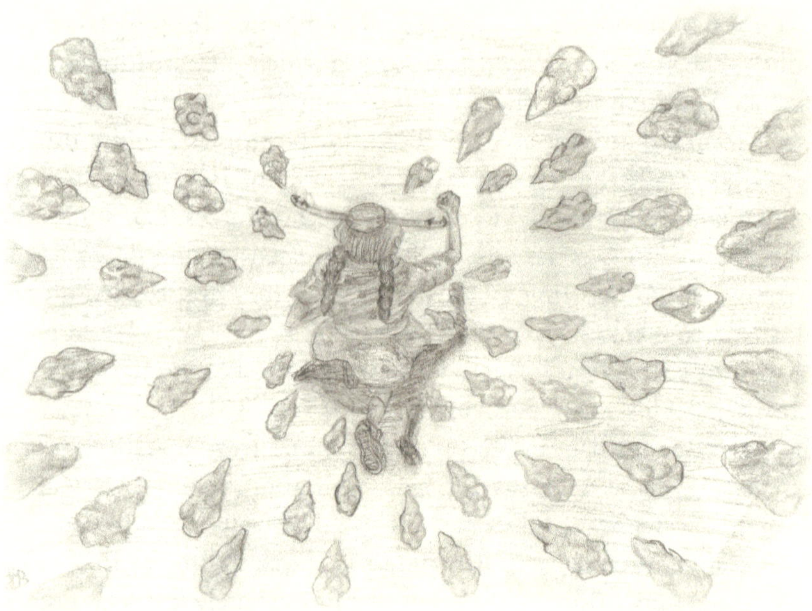

Using the dinner bell Slim rang it continuously for over one minute, which indicated to all in earshot that there was imminent danger and you should return to camp and take cover. The dinner bell is usually rung only 3 times for dinner and most everyone runs away as Cookie's cooking makes them sick. On this fateful day one camper named Sally forgot what the signal meant and took off running into a treeless area to escape Cookie's horrendous meal. What happened next was witnessed by Funny Boy who provided the following eye-witness account to the Menard County sheriff's department:

"I was standing under the solid cedar porch of the ranch house when the devil stones began to drop. I saw Sally several hundred yards off. She decided it was time to get under cover and began running at full steam toward the ranch house. There were several other ranch hands on the porch as well and we all began chanting, Go Sally Go! She did a great job of dodging right, then left, then right again. We all thought she would make it, but then, strike one—she took a hit to the shoulder and began to slow down. Then came strike two— one right on her back, then came the final blow to the head, and she was outta there! We all had to give Cassy a $5 bill as she bet that Sally wouldn't make it. What a skit this will make!"

Apparently, Sally was never good at dodgeball, and the cumulous nimbus won this round! PSL ranch hands rushed to her aid, but it was too late, Sally was stone-cold dead.

Menard County Sheriff, Buck Mueller, ruled the incident a deliberate act of revenge by Mother Nature, and that PSL Ranch was not liable for the following reasons:

1. Sally should have listened more closely to the warning bell.
2. Mother Nature cannot be held accountable in Menard County, but had this incident taken place in neighboring Concho County, they would have tried that Mother and seeded the next batch of clouds as punishment!
3. Sheriff Mueller stated he would also have chosen a knock-down if he were there, sharing in Cassy's profits.

The unfortunate bludgeoning of Sally by ice was obviously unavoidable, but all the same, PSL Ranch would like to share the following facts about hailstorms to future guests at our place in paradise:

- An estimated 1,000 soldiers died on April 13, 1360 due to a massive hail storm during the Hundred Years' War; it is known as *Black Monday*.
- Over two hundred died by hailstones during a sudden storm in the year 850 in Roopkund, India.
- In the last ten years, two Americans have been killed by hailstones.
- The largest recorded hailstone in the United States was measured at eight inches in diameter.

PSL Ranch has a warning system in place that should be taken seriously when sounded. Even if you are sickened by Cookie's meals, it is always better to side with safety and return to the ranch house when you hear the bell ringing! If you are too far away or didn't hear the bell, take cover under one of the old live oaks!

Conclusion: Don't skip gym on those days when they are playing dodgeball!

Lake Rohret Tragedy

Accidental drowning of a GTCA camper

There are many stories in old England of a lake that appears from nowhere with a beautiful spirit that rises from the depths to present a magical sword to King Arthur. This isn't one of them. Lake Rohret, which occasionally can be spotted in the center of PSL Ranch, appears periodically from one year to the next following torrential rains over the flatlands to the North. The rainwater is funneled down sloping hills and congregates in the wash to form a body of water that reaches a depth of six to twelve feet, and can remain for several months until it seeps into the limestone beneath it.

On one fateful morning, just before daybreak, a GTCA camper named Sally arose from her tent and spotted Lake Rohret for the very first time. There was a flock of ducks swimming in unison, and several axis deer on the bank sipping the cool water. Sally wanted to get closer and rolled up her jeans to enter the water. What happened next was described by Cookie who witnessed the tragedy:

"I was rockin' on the ranch house porch drinking a couple of pints of my latest brew as I was worried the Bureau of Alcohol, Tobacco, Firearms, and Explosives would find it in a raid I've been tipped off to. Anyways, I saw this camper enter the lake, and I thoughts to myself, *who would walk into the lake with all them horse crippler cactus, thorny mesquite trees, and thistles just below the surface?* Then I fell off to sleep until Slim hit me in the back of the head and asked where his breakfast was! It was a couple of hours before I remembered the incident."

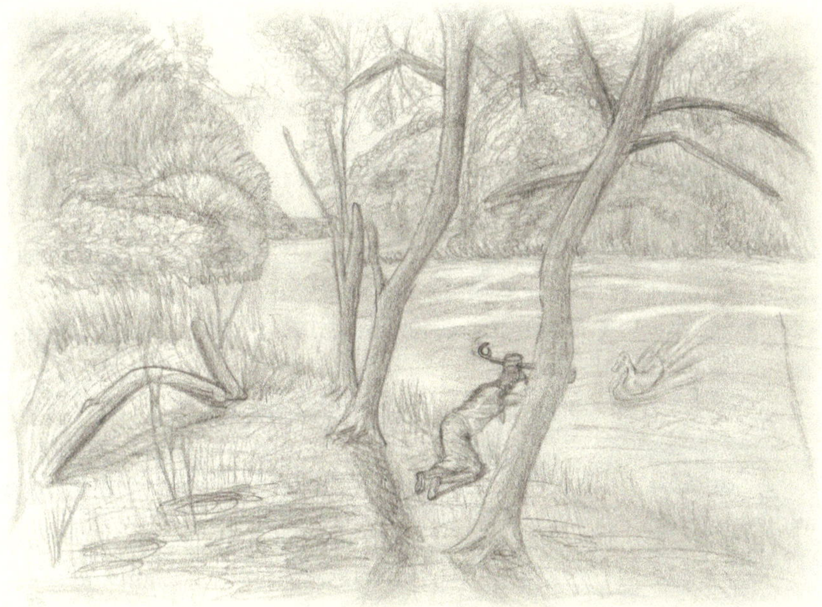

Apparently, Sally wasn't a very good swimmer, especially once her feet were filled with thorns. It appears she got caught up in some old branches and drowned in the lake. Once the GTCA camping coordinators took roll call after breakfast, it was noticed she was missing. PSL's ranch hound was called to duty, but being afraid of water, was ineffective. A search party was then organized by Cookie who found Sally floating toward the South end of the lake

Menard County Sheriff, Buck Mueller, ruled the incident an accidental drowning, and that PLS Ranch was not liable for the following reasons:

1. Sally didn't know how to swim and shouldn't have gone into the water.
2. Nobody at PSL Ranch was aware of the heavy rains up North the night before.
3. PSL Ranch had just made a contribution of $25 to his reelection campaign.

Clearly not at fault, PSL Ranch administrators nonetheless felt they should add a few facts to their visitors guide on how not to drown in Lake Rohret should it actually have water in it.

- First and foremost, don't go into the water as it is clearly not safe, or even clear for that matter.
- If you feel the urge to go in at all, wear knee high snake boots to protect you from the thorny abyss.
- Also, if you're not over 5 feet tall you will be too short and will surely drown.
- Most importantly, do not venture out alone!

Conclusion: Don't go near Lake Rohret when it actually is filled with water!

Incident #15

Bacteria—the Tiny Killer

The Feverish and Agonizing Death of a GTCA Camper

A recent study by the University of Wisconsin researchers, hereinafter referred to as Cheeseheads, has determined that farm kids have stronger immune systems than their citified peers. You see, eating a little dirt and drinking a little impure water from time to time seems to build up immunity to certain illnesses and allergies. The Cheeseheads concluded that a little bacteria and fungi unique to farm environments promote beneficially immunologic development limiting the severity of diseases and illnesses later in life (i.e., what doesn't kill you makes you stronger).

PSL Ranch is full of all types of beneficial bacteria for those raised on a farm; however, those antibiotic swallowing city kids are not so lucky! Because PSL Ranch is part of an open range. A large number of cattle droppings, known locally as cow pies, litter the landscape. In addition, the scat deposited by numerous animals, and the occasional carcass littering the property tend to taint the various water sources. Although the well on PSL Ranch contains quality water, the wash does not—even when the water seems to be clear. One GTCA camper named Sally found out the hard way that her city living would be the cause of her expiration!

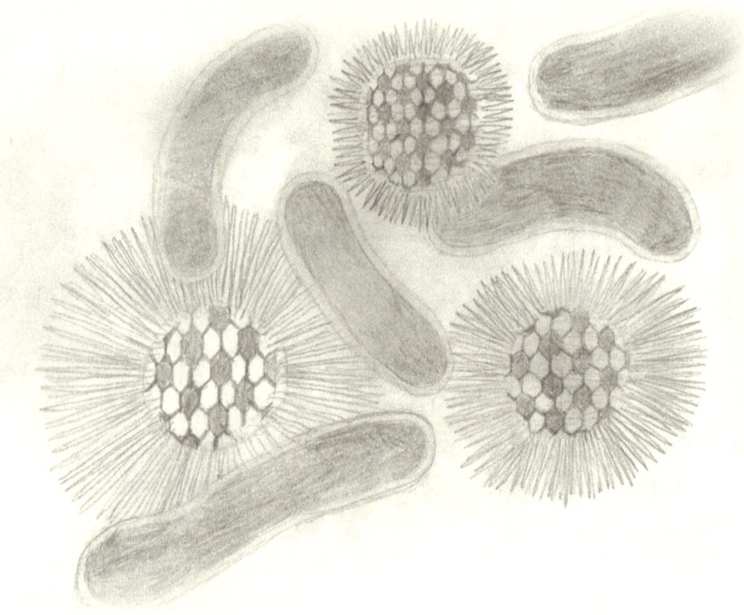

The following account of what happened to Sally was provided to the Menard County Sheriff's office by PSL Ranch's senior archeologist, Dr. S:

"I was following Shari Running Wild on one of her bow hunting expeditions to see her in action when I noticed a single camper, Sally, moving up to a pool of clear water that had settled in the middle of the wash. She was returning to camp after a long hot day of hiking and was apparently out of water.

Instead of just hiking the extra ten minutes to camp where GTCA provides bottled water, she paused, looked around, got on all fours, and began drinking. From my time in Egypt—where the water is never considered good—I knew that this was going to end badly. I don't mean Ebola bad or Black Death bad where body parts begin to rot and fall off, but more like the stomachache bad. I didn't think too much of it at the time and went on my way to witness Shari Running Wild bag a skunk for Cookie's spicy skunk soup. I went to Brady for dinner that night!"

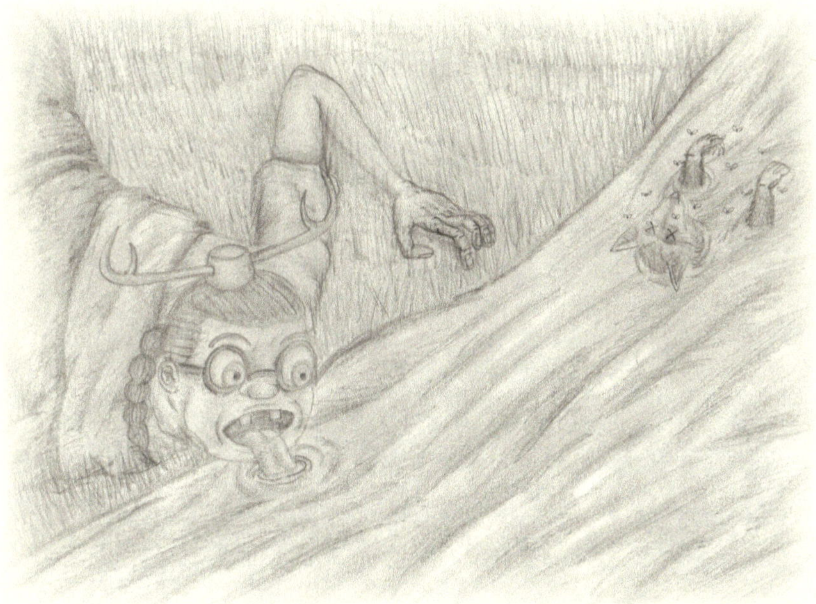

What Dr. S didn't know was that Sally was one of those kids from the city obsessed with cleanliness. She was always washing her hands, eating only fully-cooked meats, and used antibacterial soaps whenever she could. Later that night, Sally got a fever of 107 and expired on the spot. Cookie wanted to see if she could fry an egg on Sally but was discouraged by Cassy who didn't want to waste an egg.

Menard County Sheriff, Buck Mueller, ruled the incident a case of citification, and that PLS Ranch was not liable for the following reasons:

1. Sally was lazy and could have made it back to camp.
2. For any normal Menard County ranch kid, the water would not have been dangerous.
3. It was good Cookie didn't try to fry an egg as that's an old wives' tale and would have been a waste of a good egg.

PSL Ranch administrators felt just terrible about Sally's untimely departure from this world, but as those Cheesehead's pointed out; city folks just aren't that healthy and should avoid drinking tainted water. It should be noted that each year in the United States, two million people become infected with bacteria, and approximately twenty-three thousand die as a result from their infection. Many of the fatal cases are attributed to weak immune systems, or to a bacteria strain that has become resistant to antibacterial medicines due to overuse.

Conclusion: Sally is now in a better, cleaner place!

Cactuses Aren't Just Pretty Plants or Death by a Thousand Needles

Death of a GTCA Camper Due to Thousands of Cactus Needles

PSL Ranch is covered with cacti of all different kinds that provide beautiful flowers to admire and fruit for visitors to taste. The most common cactus found on the ranch flowers in multiple colors and produces a fruit named the prickly pear. Once it turns red, it can be carefully harvested and prepared in a variety of ways.

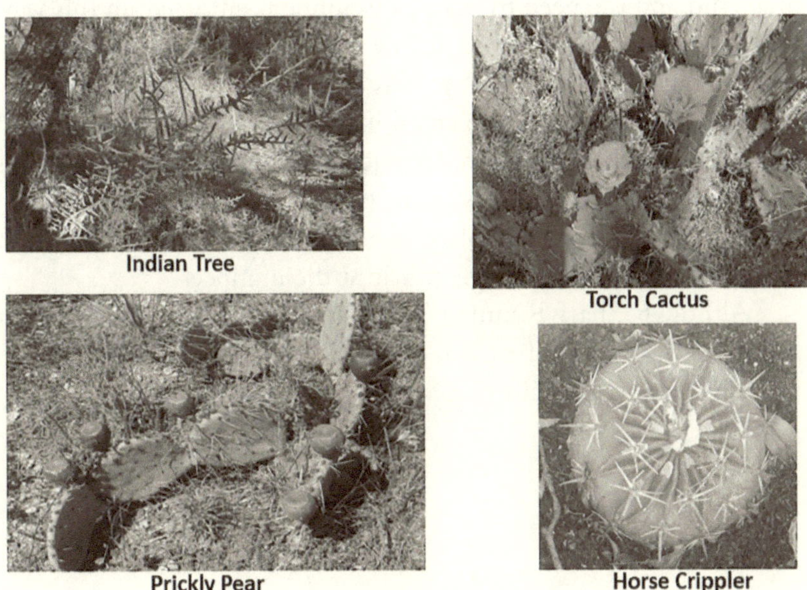

Indian Tree

Torch Cactus

Prickly Pear

Horse Crippler

Some of the cacti found on PSL Ranch

Another common cactus lies low to the ground and has very large sturdy thorns up to three inches in length. Protruding from every side, they can easily penetrate any boot that doesn't have a steel lining. These cacti are known as horse cripplers due the fact they have been known to cripple horses that step on them.

Visitors to PSL Ranch should enjoy viewing these beautiful plants, but also heed caution when walking through a cactus patch and especially handling cacti. During a mid-summer camping trip, one carefree GTCA camper named Sally had an encounter with multiple cacti while on a hike around the ranch property that didn't end well at all. The following eyewitness account is provided by Dr. S who happened to be pondering the meaning of life when the incident occurred.

Sally slept through both breakfast and the prehike briefing on the morning in question, and as far as I was concerned, she shouldn't have been allowed to go. I was overruled, as usual, by Cassy who said, "Mek di pickney gwaan, mi nah las no money!" It was no hair off my back as it was Slim who was leading the expedition, and he didn't care. He never cares about the important aspects of structure for a child and the need to ensure discipline is enforced; in this way, children learn to respect their fellow man and know how to be successful—but I digress. Anyway, Sally left the trail, grabbed a prickly pear fruit, took a bite, face planted in a patch of Indian trees, rolled over onto a batch of prickly pears, tried to get up but put both hands on a couple of horse cripplers, then rolled over on some torch cactus. I have never seen someone bleed out from so many little holes since I watched an old *Three Stooges* movie at the matinee!"

Although Shari Running Wild made it to the scene almost immediately to render first aid, she didn't have enough band aids to stop the bleeding, so Sally died.

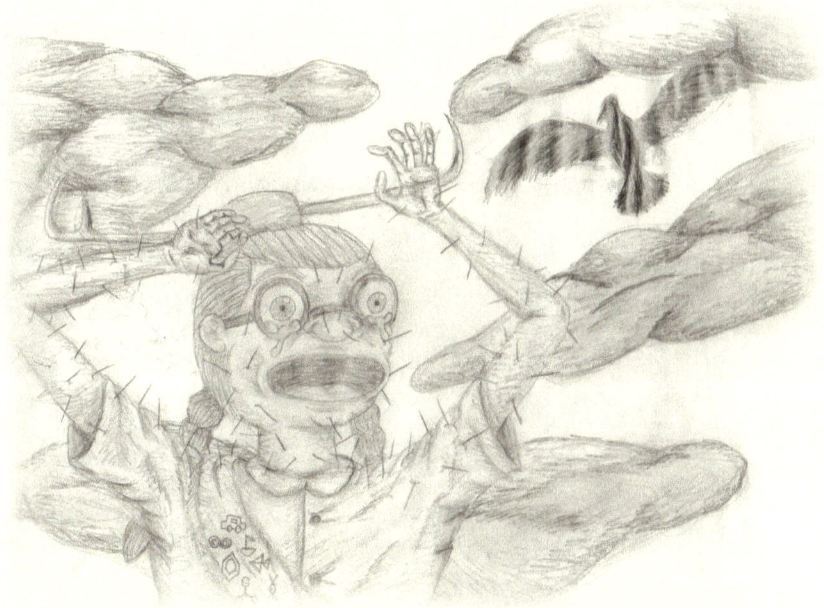

Menard County Sheriff, Buck Mueller, pointedly ruled the incident a case of misdirection, and that PLS Ranch was not liable for the following reasons:

1. Sally left the trail in the wrong direction thereby causing the accident herself.
2. Cactus cannot be charged with murder in Menard County, but had this incident taken place in Kerr County, it would have been a whole different story.
3. Lastly, and most prominently, cacti can't move; therefore, Sally had to move towards them.

It was several days before Funny Boy using his nose hair tweezers pulled enough thorns out of Sally to allow ranch hands to remove the body. During this time, it occurred to PSL Ranch authorities that a little more knowledge of the cacti that exist in this region should be provided to visitors. For instance, did you know that there are hundreds of nearly invisible thorns on a prickly pear fruit, and that you can have hundreds stuck in your fingers and hands before you ever feel them? Also, the horse crippler can penetrate an expensive pair of hiking boots before you can yell, "*ouch*!" It should also be noted that most cacti don't look like the cactus in cartoons or movies, but rather look like shrubbery or just large weeds. Basically, don't pick up any cactus or grab any plant unless you know what it is and what you are doing!

Conclusion: Don't eat prickly pear right off the cactus!

The Dancing Whitetails

Death of a GTCA Camper from a Sex-Crazed Whitetail Deer

In most states, when a deer is spotted, people take notice and admire the shy animal, which are rarely seen in the wild. Not in central Texas. These critters are all over the place and can be a nuisance at times; nor are they the docile, lovable critters that movies and cartoons make them out to be either. You see, a whitetail has a tendency to get on its hind legs and put up a fight!

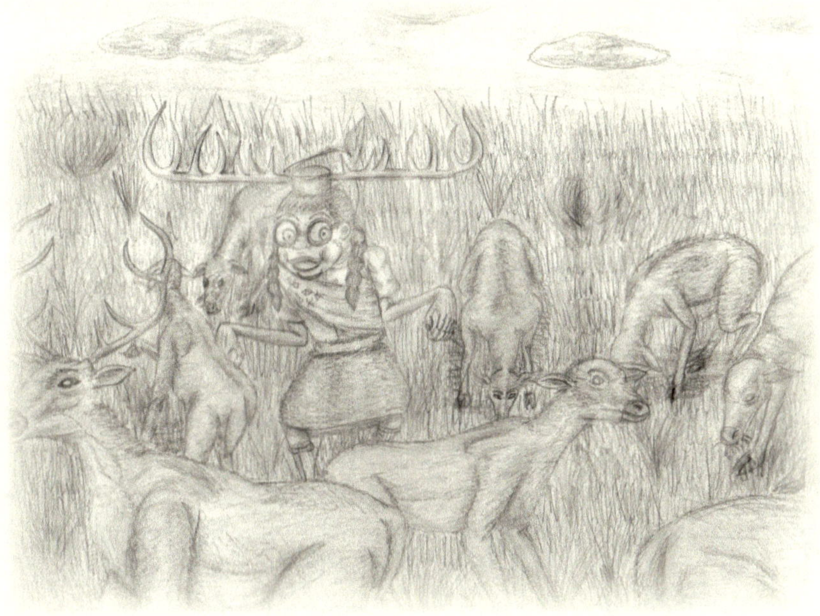

One early November morning, during the whitetail rut, a group of GTCA campers took a trip to the feeder to spot the majestic animals grazing on the free corn. The does mulling around weren't too concerned with the campers at a distance; you see, they were somewhat used to seeing an occasional GTCA member lurking around. All of a sudden, a large sixteen-point buck arrived on the scene looking for a little lovin'. One camper named Sally, who was wearing the official GTCA headdress that included a fourteen-point set of antlers, decided to pet the large buck. After all, the animated movies make them out to be so friendly!

What happened next was witnessed by Cassy, who happened to be in the area looking for a possum to cook up for the nightly BBQ:

"Mi si di pickney awalk to di deer wit one tupid at on are ed. Di deer tek are fa aneda one. It raze up on it bakfoot an beat are in are farid, an boops she ded!"

English Translation: A large whitetail buck struck Sally in the forehead, killing her instantly.

Menard County Sheriff, Buck Mueller, ruled the incident a case of mistaken identity, and that PLS Ranch was not liable for the following reasons:

1. Sally was wearing a headdress that represented a competing buck.
2. Animals can't be charged with murder in Menard County.
3. It was Sunday afternoon and he was late to his in-laws for dinner.

Obviously this incident had nothing to do with PSL Ranch, but management felt an obligation to further educate visitors on the dangers of wild beasts such as the whitetail deer.

During rut (mating season), whitetails become more aggressive and less skittish. They tend to worry more about their next date than they do about their own safety. Over fifty people are killed annually by whitetail deer in all sorts of ways, many too gruesome to mention here. In retrospect, it may not be a good idea to wear a headdress that could represent a challenge to other bucks. We at PSL Ranch approached GTCA leadership about changing their headgear to something more docile, but our request was denied.

Conclusion: Don't pet the deer!

Incident **#18**

Wild Boars: A Feral Situation

Death of a GTCA Camper from a Wild Boar Attack

Hog farms can be found all over the United States and Texas is no exception. Pigs are strong and exceptionally intelligent making them excellent escape artists. Once out of their pen they tend to run through the wildlands in groups, from several individuals to over fifty, destroying fences, crops, and just about everything else on their way to their next meal or a watering hole. With a digestive system similar to humans, in that they can eat just about anything, they are survivors and roam in large numbers over Texas ranchlands including PSL Ranch.

On an unusually hot early morning in August, near the Southend of PSL Ranch where a patch of Lake Rohret still had standing water, a GTCA camper named Sally decided to go toad hunting so she could rub them on other campers to give them warts. What happened next is provided in excruciating detail by Shari Running Wild who happened to be hugging a tree across the wash:

"Girl go wash. Scare pig. Pig kill girl"

Apparently, Sally had spooked several large hogs wallowing in what was left of Lake Rohret to stay cool. One of the larger boars, feeling cornered and threatened, charged poor little Sally, goring her to death in a gruesome example of survival instinct—something Sally lacked.

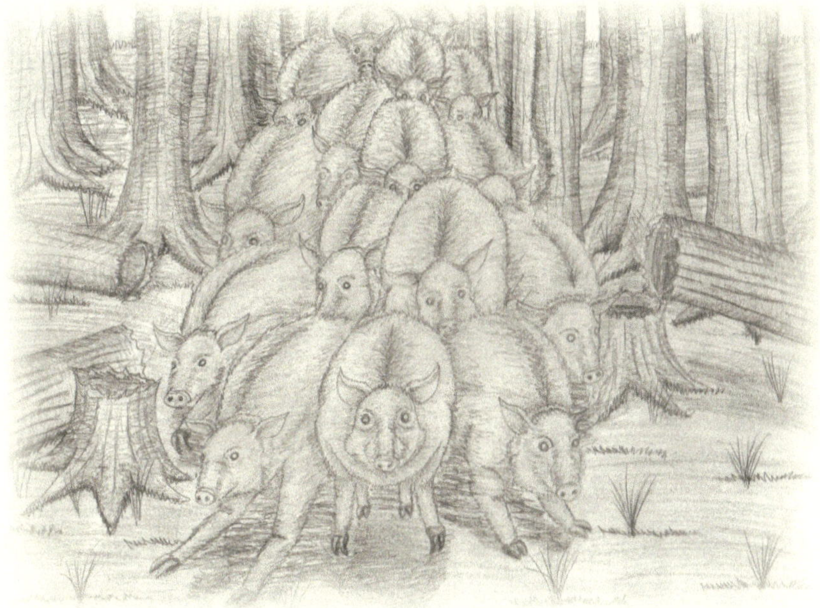

Menard County Sheriff, Buck Mueller, ruled the incident as animal abuse, and that PLS Ranch was not liable for the following reasons:

1. Sally should not have tried to give her camping companions warts by rubbing toads on them—everyone knows that's an old wives' tale.
2. Those poor pigs were just trying to stay cool and weren't bothering anyone.
3. Who hasn't seen season one of *Game of Thrones*? Sally should've known better.

We're not sure why Sheriff Mueller felt sorry for the hogs and not Sally. Perhaps he had his fill of bacon for the day. For those who haven't seen season one of the *Game of Thrones* (as unlikely as that may be), King Baratheon is mortally wounded during a hunting trip by a wild boar. These animals are large, strong, and can be aggressive when put to the test. One wild boar seen recently on PSL Ranch was estimated to weigh over five hundred pounds, and others have been spotted in the two hundred to three hundred-pound range, making them very dangerous when cornered or surprised. Even large hogs can conceal themselves under tree branches or in the shade making it easy for unsuspecting campers to walk right up to them without knowing the danger that lurks close by.

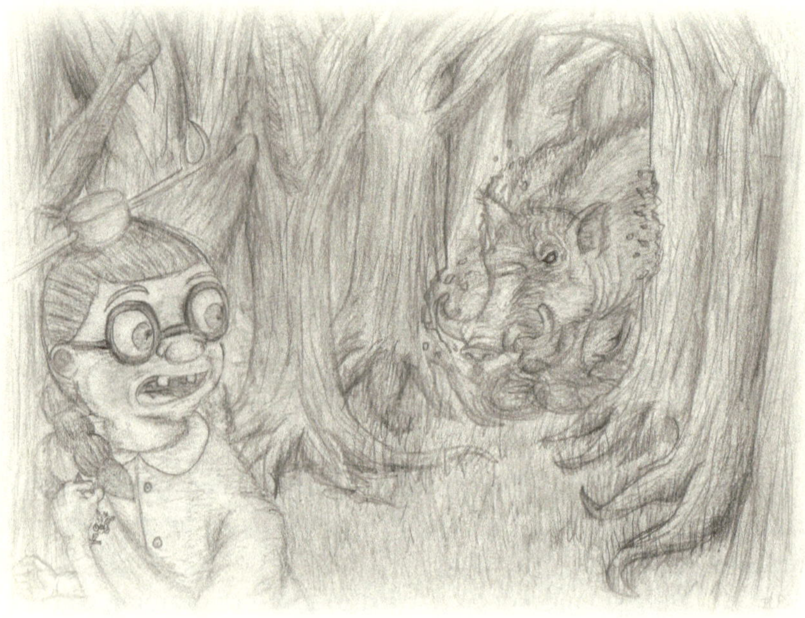

PSL Ranch hands suggest you take heed when walking in shaded areas or near the wash, particularly where the brush is high or an overhang prevents clear sight. Furthermore, if you smell fresh pig scat, it probably means there are hogs nearby! Feral hogs don't want a fight, so if you do see them don't sneak up on them; rather, make noise and watch them run away to destroy another fence line. Also, hiking in groups of two or more will further deter a hog. Only four individuals have been reportedly killed by wild hogs since 1890; not all were named Sally. It is also legal to hunt feral hogs year-round in most Texas counties as long as you have a hunting license and the hogs aren't in some farmer's pen!

Conclusion: Don't pet the pigs!

Skunk—A Smelly Situation

Death of a GTCA Camper from a Direct Spray by a Skunk

While most people run away from skunks when they spot one, Funny Boy doesn't. In fact, he has a strange passion for the small furry creatures to the point he has one for a pet. It all started several years ago when Cookie was out hunting for her famous spicy skunk soup and happened to bag the mother of a little week-old skunkette. Funny Boy took care of the little critter, feeding it and caring for it as if it were a kitten or a puppy. Now fully grown, it sits on top of his head as an ornament when he walks around the ranch. It should be noted that Funny Boy is cheap, so he never had the scent glands removed; most of the businesses in Menard refuse to let him in their stores with Ole Smelly on his head—especially since that restaurant incident two years ago!

GTCA campers love Ole Smelly, bringing treats and petting her whenever they get a chance. One GTCA camper, named Thally[3], took a liking to Ole Thmelly, and would thpend as much time around the little critter that th-he could. All the campers were briefed that the relationship between Ole Thmelly and Funny Boy wathn't normal; in fact, it wath often emphathithed that Funny Boy wathn't normal, and that Ole Thmelly juth hung around for the laughth! On one cool thpring morning at the thart of a hiking exthpedition to the far Northwethern corner of the ranch to witneth a buthard eating an

---

[3.] Sally had a speech impediment, so she pronounced her name Thally. Most of the ranch hands just thought she had a weird name and referred to her as Thally when she approached. Others spoke like she did to make her feel more at home.

old pig carcath (a favorite activity at P-Eth-L Ranch), the camperth throlled by a hollow log that happened to contain a mother thkunk and her three offthpring. Thally, being of thity hewitage and unfamiliar with the wayth of the wild, could only think of Ole Thmelly, Pepe Le Pu, and Thumper when th-he thaw the wild animal in the log and dethided to invethtigate. What happened next wath witnethed by Thhari Wunning Wild who happened to be hugging a twee upwind from the inthident:

"Girl look in log, thkunk thpray girl, girl dead."

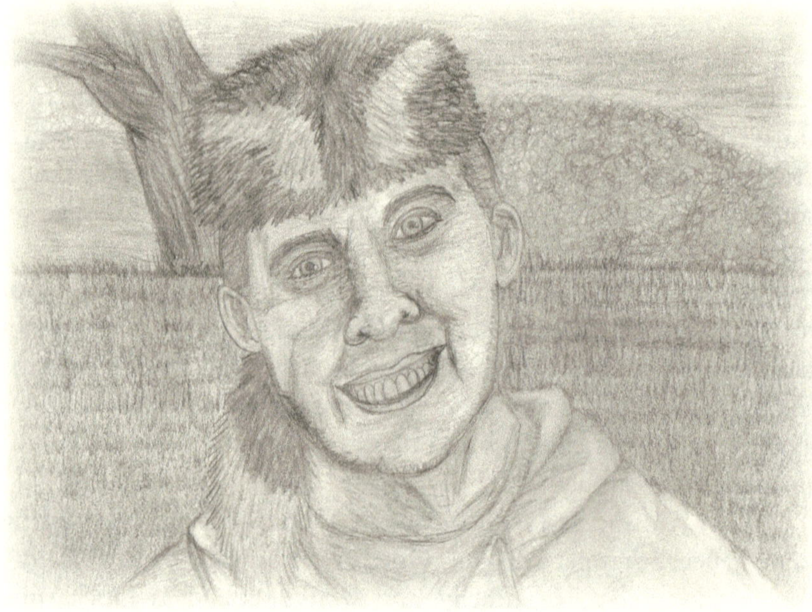

Apparentwee, Thally took the full bwunt of thpway from a larger than normal mother thkunk who wath pwotecting her young. The bwunt forthe of the sthpway went directwy into her mouth, eyeth and nothe, instantwy thutting down all bodiwy functhonth wethulting in inthant death. The other camperth, being downwind, thmelled the twagedy and wan in the oppothit dirwecthon as fath as they could. It took Thwim and Dr. Eth thwee dayths to watweeve the body uthing over five hundred gallonth of tomato juith and induthwial twath bagth. The thite now containth a hithtoweecal pwaque to mark the wocathion where *A Thinky Thkunk Thadly Thpwayed Thally.*

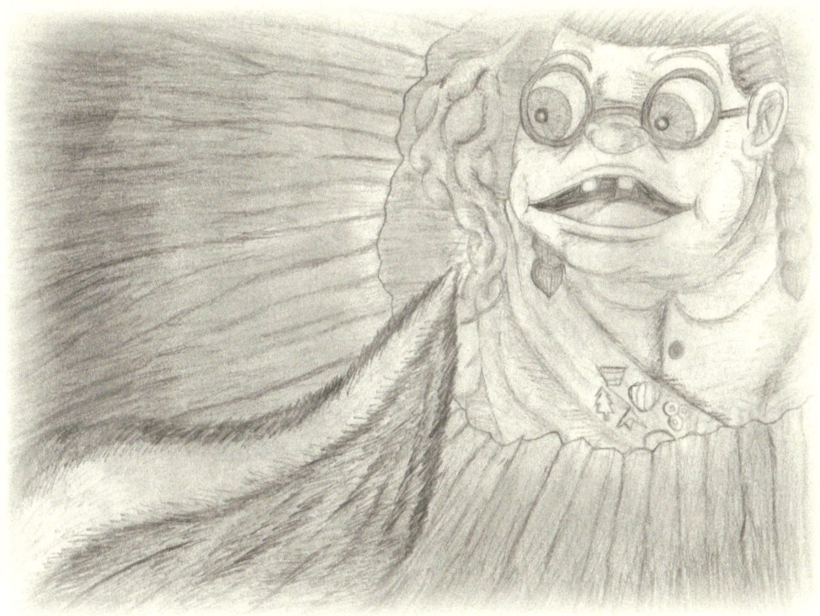

Menard County Sheriff, Buck Mueller, thought something smelled bad about this case, but eventually ruled the incident nothing more than respiratory failure and that PSL Ranch was not liable for the following reasons:

1. Thally was briefed about skunks prior to the hike and should have known better.
2. The other campers should have rendered assistance, yet they waited two hours before remembering to tell Cookie what had happened (her soup reminded them of the smell).
3. There was no one named Thally on the official PSL Ranch sign-in logs, therefore, Thally must have been a drifter.

PSL Ranch Safety Officer, Slim, decided to better educate future campers on what to expect when they come face to butt with a skunk. He now provides the following facts for visitors to our paradise in the sun:

- Skunk spray is so potent that it can kill you.[4]
- Skunks nest in shelters built by other animals, in hollow logs, or abandoned buildings.
- Female skunks give birth to as many as ten young each year.
- Skunks are nocturnal feeders that eat about everything and will invade your camp when they smell food.
- Wild skunks do not make good pets, but will become "friendly" when fed; just ask Shari Running Wild next time you see her!

We hope any confusion over whether skunks should be treated as pets is now clear. To keep all that tomato juice from going to waste, Cookie prepared a large pot of Spicy Skunk Soup in memory of Thally's passing!

Conclusion: Don't pet the skunks!

---

4. http://voices.nationalgeographic.com/2014/03/11/skunks-spray-evolution-animals-science/.

Lightning or Death from Above!

Inappropriate Attempt to Harness Energy by a GTCA Camper

Texas is known for its ferocious storms, and people come to watch and chase storms as a pastime. Lightning is a common occurrence, even when there is only a single storm cloud in the skies above. Our rapidly moving warm and cold fronts provide light spectacles that can't be beat, but there are precautions you should take in a lightning storm to prevent injury or death. Professional storm chasers know when they should take cover as do most Texans who have lived with storms all their lives.

On one warm spring day, a group of GTCA campers from New York were just finishing a morning hike when the winds shifted to the North and it began to rapidly cool down. Thunderheads began building overhead, and it wasn't long before everyone could hear Cassy yelling, "Keep yuself still—nu mek lightning ketch yu!" The returning hikers looked puzzled at her comment and kept on going to watch the storm. One camper, Sally, had just received a pair of new golf shoes for a trip to the Menard Golf course the next day and wanted to break them in. They were top-of-the-line with half-inch steel spikes for better balance when swinging a three iron. As the other hikers slowly returned to the ranch house, Sally could be seen running back and forth in a pasture trying out her new shoes.

What happened next was witnessed by Slim who provided the following testimonial to the Menard County sheriff's department:

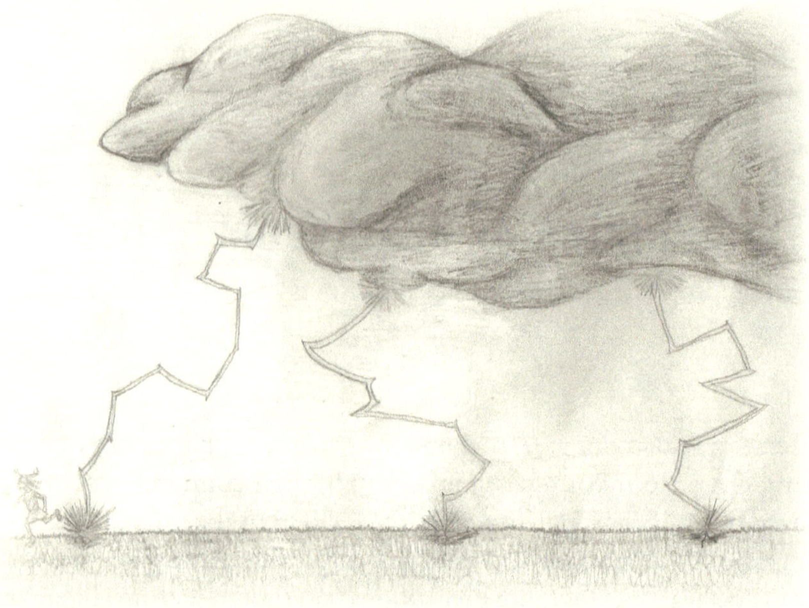

"I heard Cassy give a warning about lightning and went out to take a look at the storm. I saw the hikers coming towards the ranch house; all but one who was running around all odd-like and occasionally pretending to swing somethin'. I was about to saddle a horse and ride out to see what was what when I remembered we don't have a horse. It was then that I heard an awful loud crack and I sees that little camper girl lit up like a light bulb! As I began to walk toward the area where I thoughts the lightning struck, I sees her git up, smoking a little, and start wabblin' my way. I was happy as she was going to make it when a second bolt got her again! Funny, I always thoughts that lightning didn't strike twice in the same spot! Anyways, when I got there she was crispy and dead."

Apparently, Sally's steel spikes provided the grounding necessary for the storms electrical discharge to find a connection… twice!

Menard County Sheriff, Buck Mueller, ruled the incident as two acts of God, and that PSL Ranch was not liable for the following reasons:

1. Cassy had provided the warning telling the hikers to return to the ranch house.
2. Sally was mostly at fault wearing those silly shoes.
3. God must have really wanted Sally dead, striking her twice, and who am I to take issue with God!

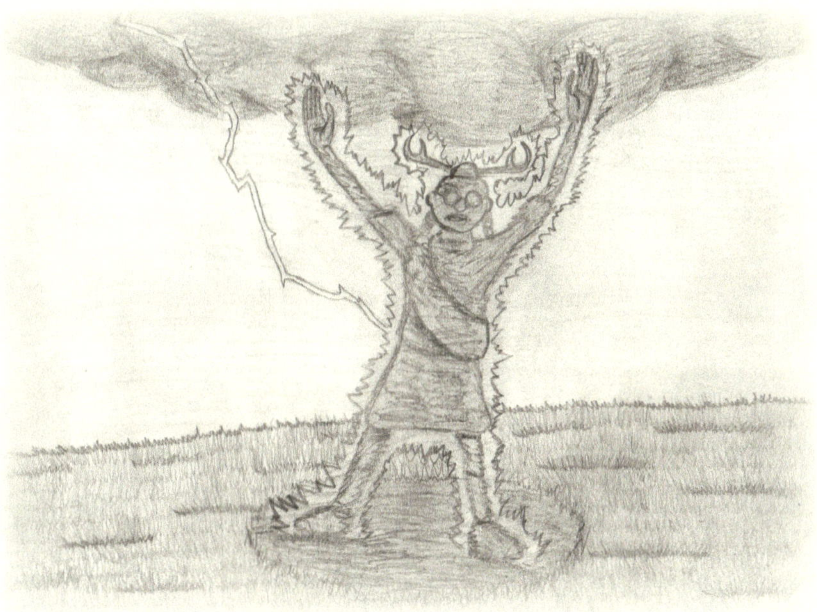

Once Cassy quit laughing, she felt bad and decided to add some facts about lightning to the PSL Ranch Safety manual to include:

- Over fifty people are killed by lightning annually in the United States.
- Only 10 percent of those struck by a lightning bolt die.
- Texas has more lightning deaths than any other state.
- Lightning hates golfers.
- A lightning bolt is only about one inch in diameter.

- Lightning usually only strikes a location once, but not always.

The golf tournament in Menard was a success and was held in Sally's honor. The trophy given to the top golfer was renamed, Sally's Bolt.

Conclusion: Don't golf in a lightning storm!

The Dorothy Effect (Tornado)

Disappearance of a GTCA camper

We've discussed several types of Central Texas weather so far: wind, hail, and lightning, but not the most destructive weather phenomenon, tornados. Every year, thousands of people and numerous communities are affected by the more than 150 mph circular winds that rip apart buildings and toss vehicles hundreds of yards during short, violent periods of destruction. PSL Ranch has been lucky as the size of many of our old live oak trees indicate that there has not been a tornado, at least recently, on our ranch property causing damage. Still, it's always a good idea to keep a close ear to radio announcements whenever a storm rolls through.

One late spring afternoon, a series of large storms began moving into Central Texas. These rapidly moving storms were reportedly accompanied by heavy rain and large hail. Due to a previous incident (#13) where a GTCA camper was lethally attacked by large devil stones, PSL Ranch administrators decided to call all campers into the ranch house as a precaution.

Earlier that day, the campers were in an open area near the ranch house having fun with dust devils. Dust devils are small columns of circular winds that sometimes occur during clear skies. They kick up dust and look like a baby tornado, but are mostly harmless and fun to run through if you're close enough to do so. As the day went on and the storms rolled through, Slim began ringing the bell continuously as he spotted a small funnel cloud descending from the tail-end of the storm. What happened next was witnessed by Cookie who provided the following report to the Menard County sheriff's department:

"I was tossin' out the remains of my famous dead critter soup when I noticed a couple of GTCA campers runnin' out the back of the ranch house toward what they thought was a large dust devil. Once I finished scrapin' out the chunks stuck on the bottom of the pot, which nobody wanted anyways, I moseyed back out to take another look. By this time the twister had grown in size and the campers were running back to the ranch house as fast as they could. I thought they would make it back safely, but one of them, Sally I think her name was, turned to the right directly in the twister's path! It grabbed her, and she begun going in circles around and around and around. I got so dizzy watching I passed out for a bit, and when I wakes up, both the camper and the twister were gone!"

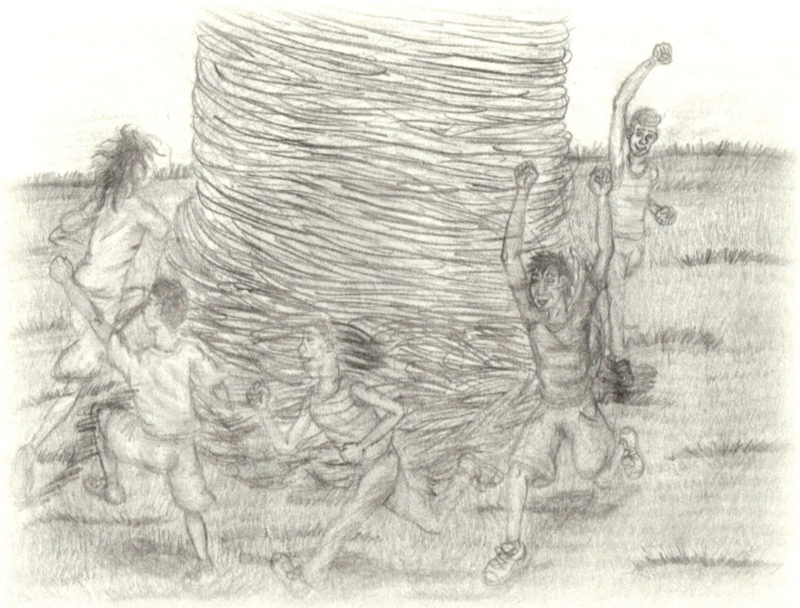

Apparently, the F2 tornado that rolled through Menard County just did a touch-n-go after it captured Sally in its winds. The storm rapidly moved out of the area, and Sally was never seen again.

Menard County Sheriff, Buck Mueller, ruled the incident a blustery event, and PSL Ranch not liable for the following reasons:

1. Slim sounded the alarm early and called the campers into the ranch house.
2. Sally and the other campers snuck out on their own.
3. Since she couldn't be found, it's safe to assume Sally is safe and sound in Oz!

Worried about future businesses from GTCA, PSL Ranch administrators decided to provide the following facts about dust devils and tornados to prevent future incidents involving possible trips to Oz:

Dust devils are mostly harmless but have been known to be large enough to cause damage to people and property.

A *dust devil* is a strong, long-lived whirlwind. A Whirlwind usually lasts for only a few seconds.

- Dust devils often occur when the skies are clear.
- On average, there are about one thousand tornados each year.
- Approximately eighty people are killed by tornados each year in the United States.
- During a forty-seven-year period, 1,550 tornados were recorded in Texas, killing 865 people, or an average of 18.4 deaths annually.
- Most deaths occur due to flying debris.

We hope these facts will calm the fears of anyone wanting to visit our Central Texas version of the Garden of Eden. After all, Dorothy's experience in Oz wasn't all bad!

Conclusion: Don't play with tornados!

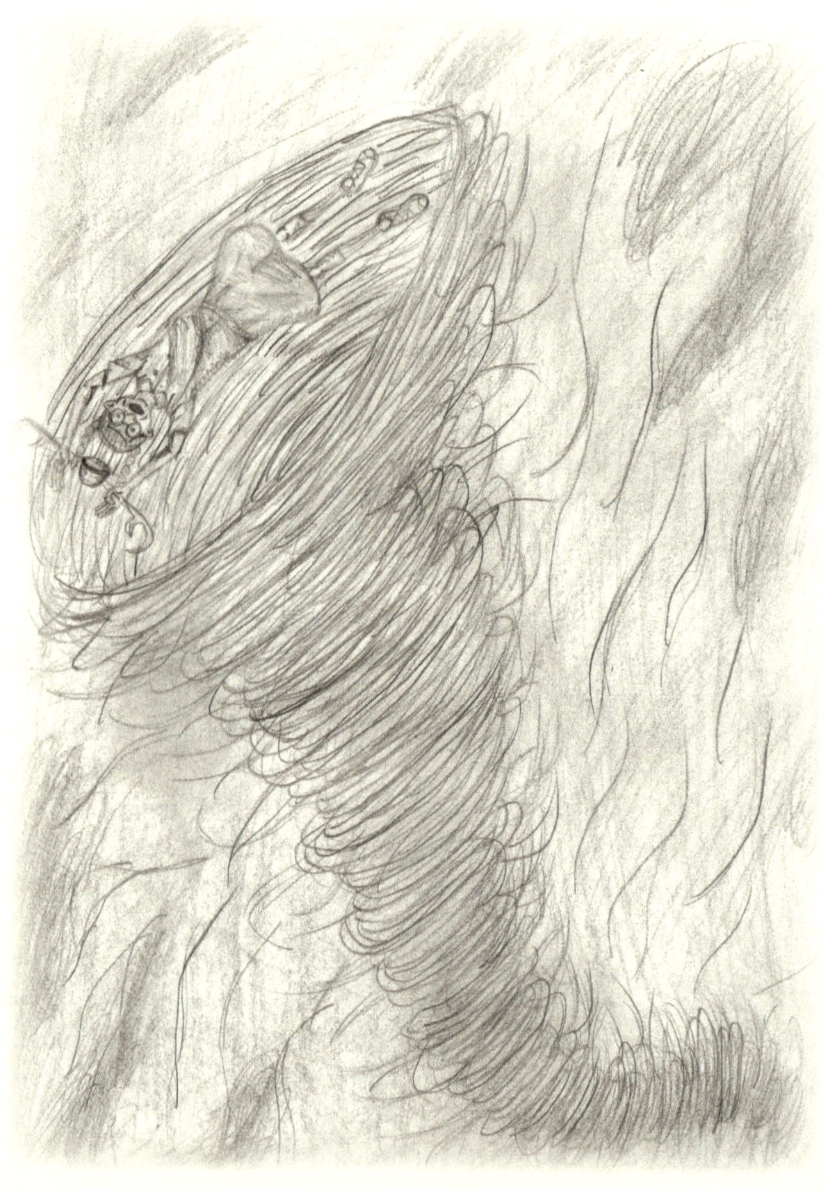

Hunting Season: A Texas Pastime
The Accidental Shooting of a GTCA Camper

Texans take their hunting seasons very seriously as many are out to get a trophy whitetail to mount on their cabin wall. Bragging rights are important, and deer season opens thirty minutes before the official sunrise making it sometimes difficult to see the finer details of the quarry a hunter may be aiming at.

In early November on the first day of hunting season, an out-of-state hunter named Dick Chainy was sitting in his leased deer blind twenty feet above the ground, spying the area surrounding a feeder on PSL Ranch. This feeder was dispersing corn several times a day to attract wildlife to make it easier for campers to view them in their unnatural habitat. The following testimonial from PSL Ranch hand Shari Running Wild provides a detailed eyewitness account of Sally's final moments.

"Sally go feeder. Sally run around deer. Sally git shot."

Menard County Sheriff, Buck Mueller, ruled the shooting accidental and PSL Ranch not liable for the following reasons:

1. The GTCA official uniform included a hat with a fourteen-point antler on top.
2. It was foggy the morning of the incident.
3. Following the shooting, Mr. Chainy correctly tagged and field-dressed Sally per Texas State Hunting Regulations.

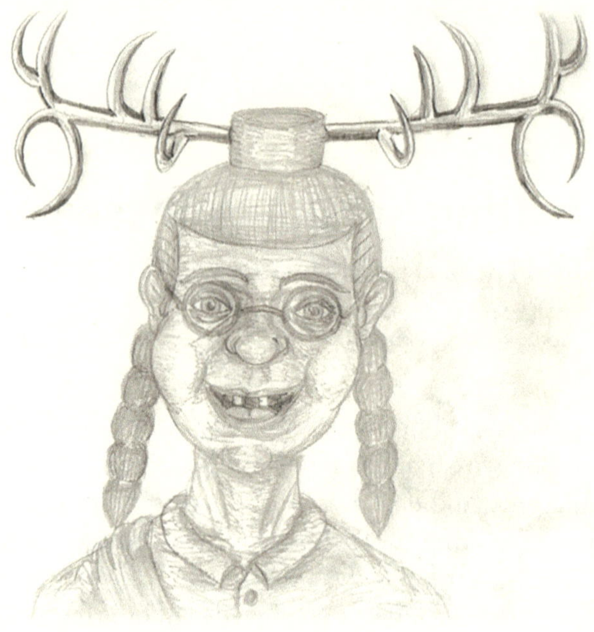

Mr. Chainy was allowed to keep and mount his quarry. His fourteen-point trophy is said to be proudly displayed on his living room wall.

Preventive actions have been taken by PSL Ranch administrators to minimize the possibility of future incidents of this nature. Future GTCA headgear is now required to only display the antlers of a spike. This will prevent adult hunters from accidently shooting a camper as only minors can harvest spike bucks. Furthermore, it is unlikely anyone would want to mount and display a spike on their cabin wall.

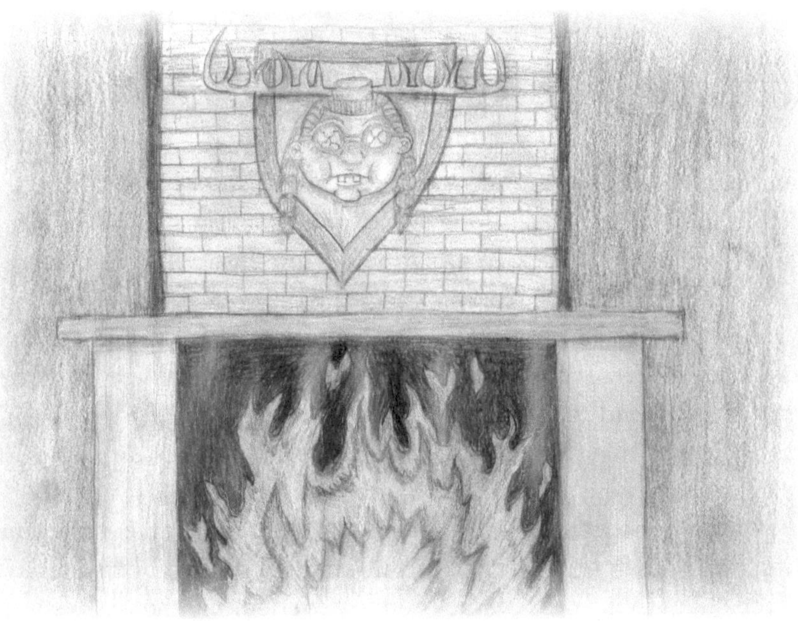

Conclusion: Guns don't kill people, politicians with guns do!

<h1 style="text-align:center">INCIDENT #23</h1>

Dirty Feet: Death by Jamaican!
Death of a GTCA Camper due to a Broken Neck

When Cassy and Slim purchased the remote property now known as PSL Ranch, it was a wild place filled with every type of cactus and thistle that grows in central Texas. This includes mesquite trees, brush, and critters that slither and fly just waiting to bite or sting you—sending you back to where you came from. The Sun blazed down on the landscape making it feel like they were in an oven. They realized that if you were in need of help there was no one there to assist, lest it was the survivalist couple over on yonder range, but even they didn't spend much time in this harsh and unforgiving environment. It was an open, untamed, and unforgiving Texas range with roaming cattle and aboriginals that crept around day and night.[5]

Well not a hell of a lot has changed since then, except the construction of the ranch house; an 1860's timber cabin set between two of the oldest living oaks on the property overlooking the wash (sometimes referred to as Lake Rohret). Cassy and Slim put their blood and sweat in building this cabin, mostly standing around watching a log stacker do all the work, but it was their pride and joy once it was finished. Cassy spent much of her time each day cleaning and making the new cabin the center piece of PSL Ranch. In fact, she was obsessed with keeping it in new condition and only took breaks to torment Slim with voodoo magic, or to hunt possums for Cookie's evening meals.

---

[5] The term *aboriginals* in this context refers to local contractors looking for work.

One rare rainy day, Cassy was inside polishing the natural cedar floors until they sparkled. All of the ranch hands knew better than to tread upon this sacred space lest they be severely beaten about the head and neck. Unfortunately, one GTCA camper named Sally found out the hard way. The following testimonial was provided to the Menard County sheriff's department by Cassy in excruciating and unintelligible detail:

"Mi did leave di door open to mek di floor dry a likkle bit; an mi a-look pon di beautiful shine, when dat damn Sally come inna di ouse wid ar dutty shoes. She did plan to teef some a Cookie raccoon chip biscit. Mi was just tinkin, 'A whe Cookie de, ar biscit a bun up!' when dis rude pickney se to mi, 'A whe di biscit ole woman!' Well, dat was di las straw. Mi las mi mine… grab up di pickney and trow ar ova di railling! Mus e a ten-foot drop. A tink di las time mi so vex was when Slim did buy dis ya lan! Well, mi a cleanup did pickney mess fi bout twenty minute, when mi did ear Shari Runnin Wile se, 'Sally fall, Sally dead,' a so it go. Mi awright now, but mi did kill di gal pickney… so arres mi, offisa!"

English Translation: ???

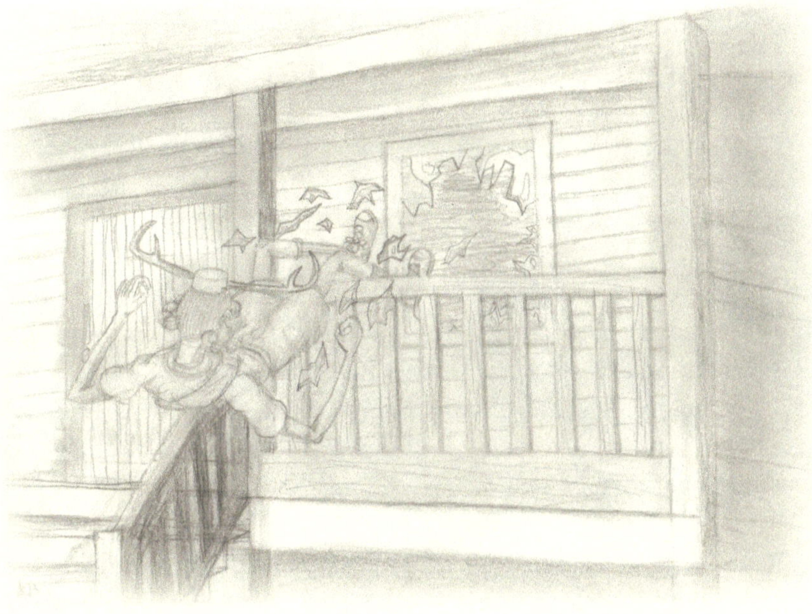

Menard County District Attorney, Toyoto Ahslc… Achwl… Ms. T, was becoming mighty suspicious of PSL Ranch following her review of this incident and asked Menard County's District Judge, Rob Hangman, to request an official police sketch to help determine liability. The Honorable Rob Hangman, lamenting that the last hanging in Menard County occurred on 23 December 1878, was all too happy to oblige and ordered Sheriff Mueller to comply. Sheriff Mueller, not having a budget for a sketch artist, accomplished the drawing himself.

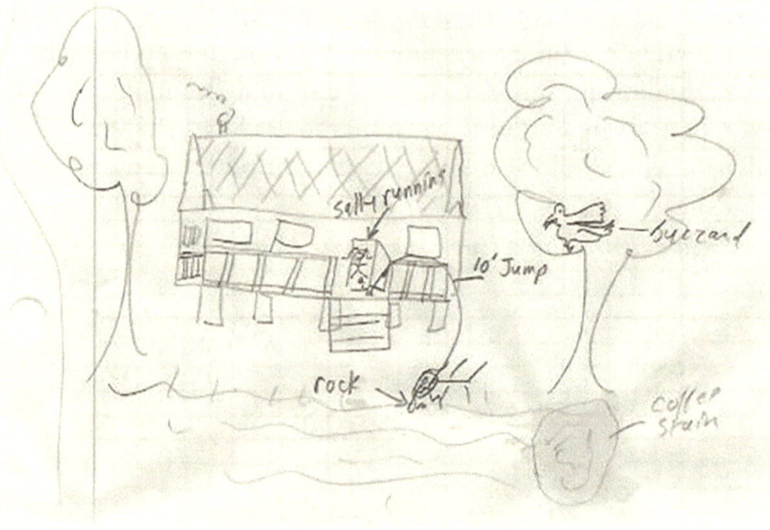

After careful review and a pint of Cookie's confiscated home brew, it was clear to Ms. T that this incident was in no way PSL Ranch's fault, calling off any further investigation.

Therefore, Menard County Sheriff, Buck Mueller, ruled Sally's death a self-inflicted accident, and that PSL Ranch was not liable for the following reasons:

1. Cassy's explanation of what happened was unintelligible, and therefore, could not be used as evidence in a court of law.

2. Sally's footprints ended five feet from the ledge indicating she must have leaped over the side, landing on one of the large rocks below.
3. Sally should have used the steps.

PSL Ranch administrators feel mighty bad about this… accident and would like to alert campers and other visitors of several other misappropriate actions that could send Cassy into such a rage. You see, Cassy used to be a champion power-lifter and can still toss a small child a very long way!

Other issues that may end up shortening your life in the PSL Ranch house:

*   Sitting on furniture while wearing dirty clothes; if you must sit for a bit, take a log by the fire pit
*   Splashing or spilling water on the cabin's cedar floors—and not cleaning it up!
*   Making a mess in the kitchen and not cleaning it up
*   Making a mess anywhere in the ranch house and not cleaning up after yourself
*   Not immediately adhering to Cassy's commands (just ask Slim!)

Conclusion: Wipe your feet before entering the ranch house!

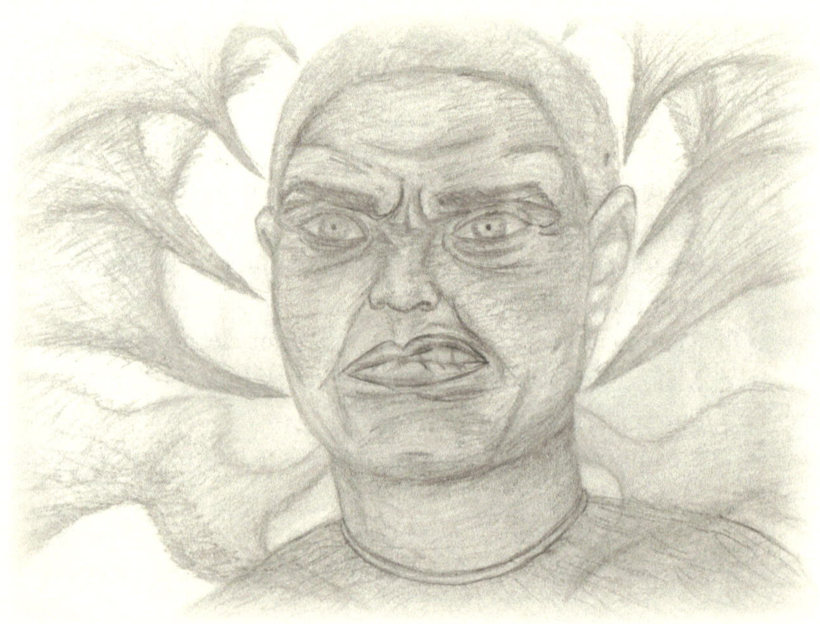

Wildfire: As Fast as the Wind
The BBQ Death of a GTCA Camper

Burn bans are in effect most of the year in Menard and surrounding counties for a good reason—it's dry! Annual rainfall is around twenty-four inches, and most of it comes in the spring, leaving the vegetation dry the other three seasons. In the late afternoon wind gusts up to twenty-five miles per hour, greatly increasing the chance a campfire can get out of control, so precautions must be taken to prevent range fires. Starting in early November, hunters from all over the United States and other countries congregate in Central Texas for our famous whitetail deer hunts, and many of these hunters don't have a clue about the hazards.

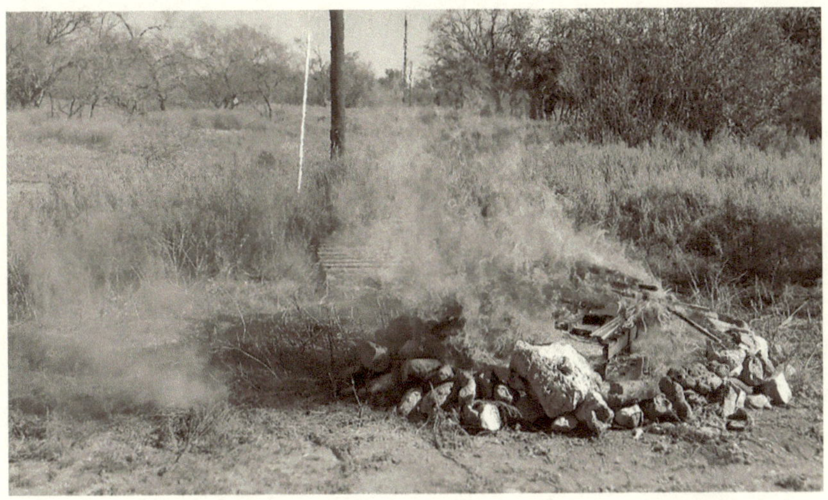

One of Cookie's campfires nearly getting out of control!

On a seasonably warm November afternoon, a group of GTCA campers were on PSL Ranch's Eastern boundary chasing jack rabbits with sticks (not a nice thing to do) when suddenly a strong breeze picked up from the South. It was then that several of the campers smelled smoke, and it wasn't from campfire wood or the wood-burning stove, but instead had a pungent smell that included weeds and grass. All the campers sensed danger and began running back to the ranch house except one, Sally, who wanted to knock one more jack rabbit in the head before returning to safety. What happened next was witnessed by Dr. S who provided the following statement to Menard's volunteer fire department:

"I was investigating an Indian burial mound recently discovered on PSL Ranch. It turned out that it was just a hole Shari Running Wild used to bury Cookie's food so the animals wouldn't eat it and get sick. I smelled the grassfire and started quickly back to the campsite where we have water and fire extinguishing equipment to combat these types of fires. It was then I looked up to see a silhouette of a camper, Sally I think, running in circles with a stick trying to whack something while a range fire rapidly approached behind her! What kind of kid would hit innocent animals in the head for fun? This is a result of a child with non-participating parents in her life, leaving her to devise ways to entertain herself when she should be having quality family time… but I digress; anyway, before she knew it, the fire had encircled her and she was no more."

Apparently, Sally's urge to hit large-headed rabbits in the noggin was greater than her urge to flee from danger, and the fire consumed her. Wildfires on an open range travel nearly as fast as the wind, which can easily overtake a human fleeing for their life.

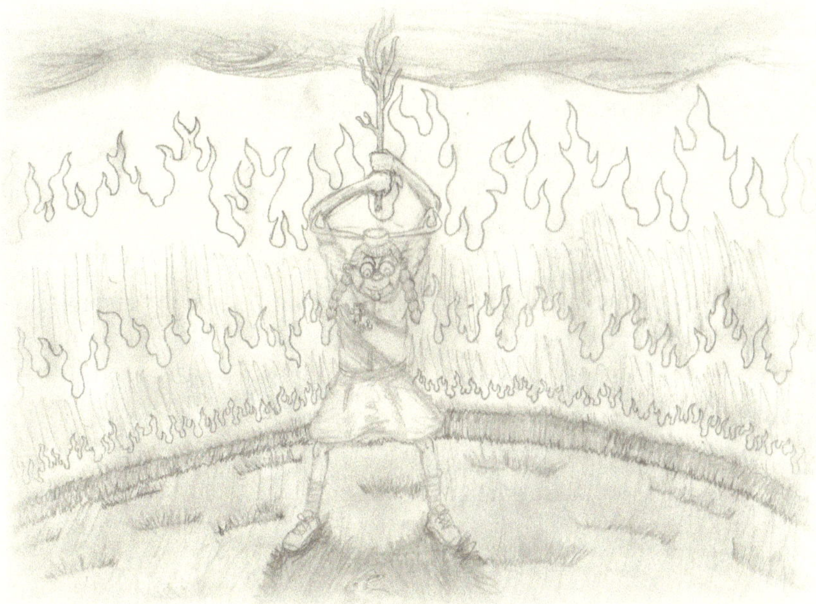

Menard County Sheriff, Buck Mueller, rubbed a burn scar on his left leg and lamented the days he used to whack jack rabbits. He then ruled the incident as an act of Darwinism and that PSL Ranch was not liable for the following reasons:

1. Whacking rabbits in the noggin is only allowable if the whacker has a Texas hunting license, and Sally did not.
2. Sally should have heeded the warning signs; to include everyone else was fleeing and screaming, and the mile-long line of roaring flames heading her way.
3. The fire did not start on PSL Ranch property.

PSL Ranch's fire marshal, Cassy, felt mighty bad about the unintentional crisping of Sally and now educates newly arrived visitors with some facts about wildfires:

- Wildfires kill 339,000 people annually worldwide; 157,000 in sub-Saharan Africa alone!

- Smoke inhalation is the greatest cause of death from a wildfire.
- Most deaths in the United States are in rural areas where early warning is not available or are a direct result of attempting to fight the fire, where a change in wind can entrap firefighters.

Although the smell of barbecue hung in the air for several days following this incident, we at PSL Ranch feel the danger of a similar fatality is low and shouldn't prevent anyone from visiting God's Country.

Conclusion: Don't whack the rabbits!

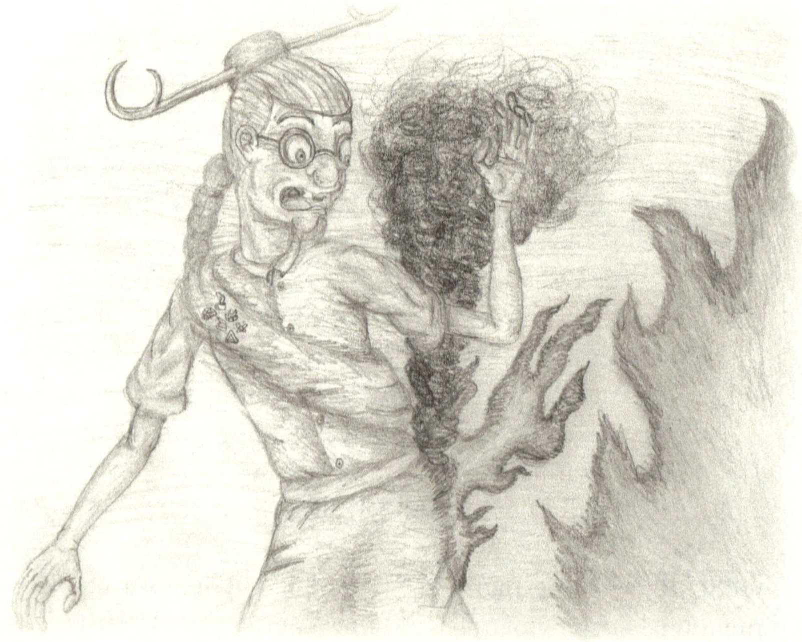

The Rapids—A Rare Event!

Death of a GTCA Camper Due to Extreme Sports

There are many exciting adrenaline-pumping sports and adventures on PSL Ranch and our visitors routinely partake in many of these activities. They include running away from the cattle, running away from rattlesnakes, running away from rabid animals, running away from cougars, running away from skunks, running away from wild-fires, and of course, running away from Cookie's cooking!

One extreme sport PSL administrators strongly recommend against while visiting our Ranch is attempting to kayak our level 5 rapids. There are several good reasons for not attempting to kayak down our rapids: they're dry most of the time, the only method of navigating them is with our lake kayaks, and on the rare occasion water is rushing down the rapids into calmer water—they are unpredictable and unsafe.

On one rare occasion, a perfect storm occurred in Northern Menard and surrounding counties, which provided an opportunity for an adrenaline junkie GTCA camper named Sally to attempt the rapids for the very first time. Sally was from far Northwest Texas (some call it Colorado) and thought the local area to be boring. She had heard tales around the campfire about how the rapids appear for no reason and run for hours before vanishing—even when the skies were clear! On this evening, the GTCA campers were on an expedition to view the stars during a new moon when they suddenly heard rushing water. This seemed odd since the skies above were clear and the wind calm. Sally ran to the Northernmost location on PSL Ranch and saw what looked like a raging river pouring directly into a rapidly filling Lake Rohret! She took a kayak off the rack and ran back to the rapids. Cookie, who was leading the expedition that evening, yelled in a quiet monotone voice, "No, stop, don't do it," and then took another swig of homemade brew from a mason jar. What happened next was witnessed by Cassy who took the rapids as a bad omen:

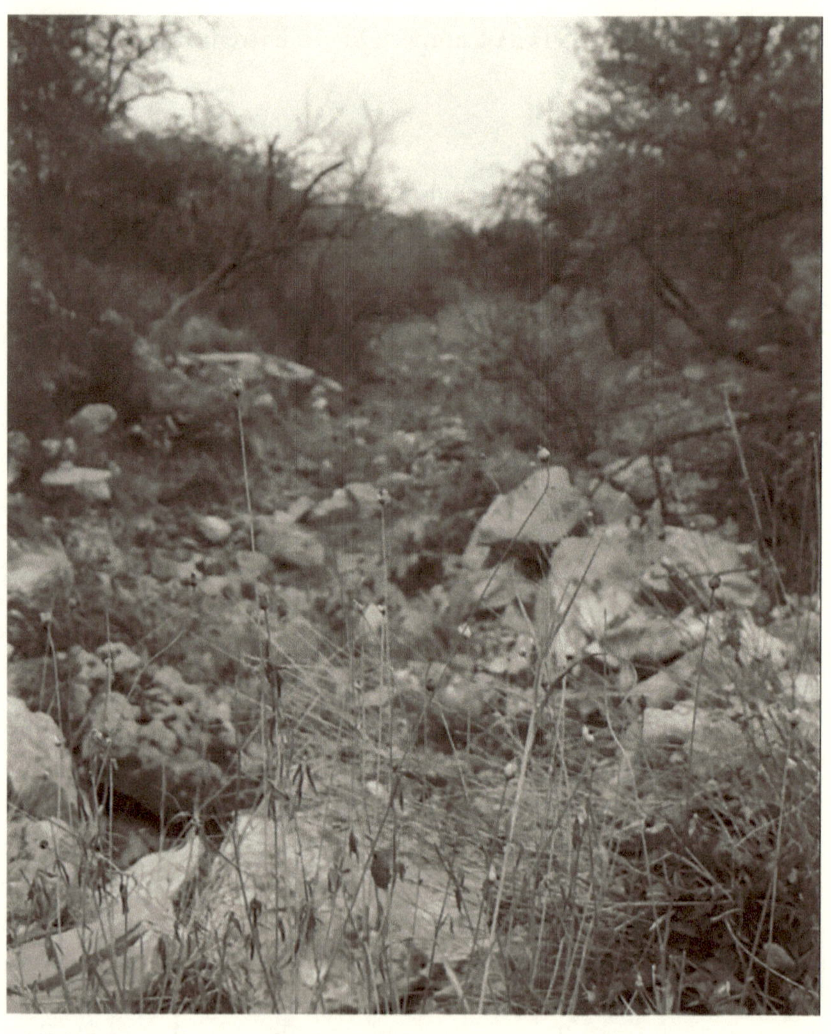

PSL Rapids, in a dry state!

"Mi si di pickney tect di boat an pushit inna di wata at di top a di wash. Two a dem go down, but only one a dem come up. Mi neva ear are cry out, so she mussy dead."

English Translation (provided by Slim): I witnessed Sally taking a kayak from the rack without permission and head up to the top of the rapids. With the oar in her hands, she pushed off the side of the bank gingerly into the rushing waters as one would normally do. Cookie was yelling frantically for her to stop, but Sally gave no heed and continued down the eight-foot waterfall into the churning waters below! After a brief moment, the kayak shot up out of the torrent of frothing water, but Sally was nowhere to be seen. After an exhaustive search by the entire PSL Ranch community over the following days, Sally's body could not be found, and sadly, the search was called off.

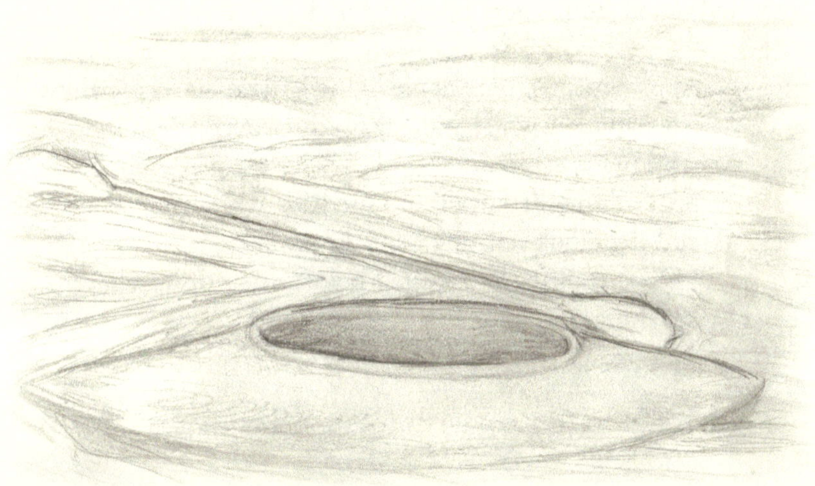

Menard County Sheriff, Buck Mueller, ruled the incident as another missing person's report and PSL Ranch not liable for the following reasons:

1. PSL ranch hand Cookie correctly sounded the alarm.
2. Sally initiated the extreme sport on her own without consulting other camp officials.
3. There was no body, therefore no crime or misconduct to report.

To prevent further such incidents, PSL Ranch officials have clearly marked *no kayaking* at the location of the rapids with a three-by-five index card nailed to a tree. We hope this discourages future adrenaline junkies from attempting such a dangerous feat. To further discourage such attempts, the following information is now provided in the initial ten-hour safety briefing for all new campers:

- Approximately ten people in the United States die annually from guided white water kayaking; over one hundred die worldwide.
- Specially made kayaks are used for white water kayaking, and they look nothing like lake kayaks.
- Special training is required before attempting white water kayaking.

Either Sally didn't know the risks involved, or she was just plain stupid. But to this day, fishermen and kayakers on the San Saba River at Cowboy Hole, where the wash empties, say they see a ghost kayaker in the late evening asking for directions back to PSL Ranch!

Conclusion: Don't kayak at PSL Ranch!

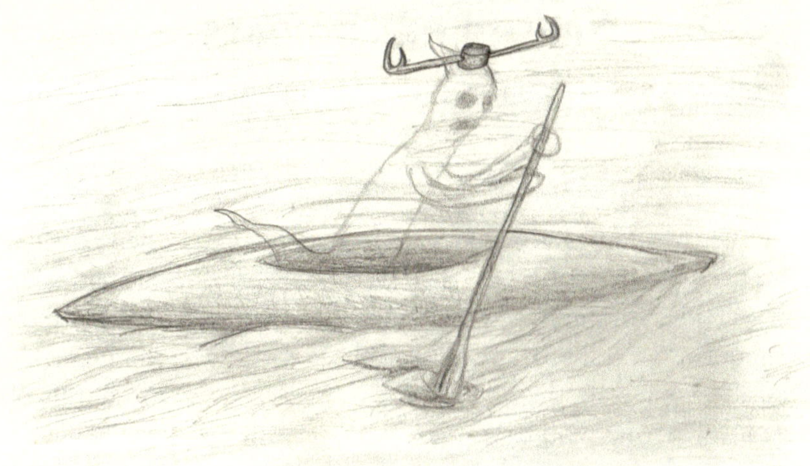

Trespassing Means Open Season on Campers

Death of a GTCA Camper Due to an Illegal Maneuver

There are two things newcomers immediately notice when traveling on central Texas rural roads, that every rancher or local that passes you will give a friendly wave and that *no tresspassing* signs are more numerous than the buzzards overhead. As friendly as the locals are, they also appreciate their privacy! A lot has to do with the out-of-state hunters who tend to trounce over everyone's property as if they own it. With the remote homesteads, open ranges, and cattle herds roaming around, you can understand why those living in this quiet community get a little unnerved when they see strangers with guns sneaking about. The effect on homesteader's nerves from those nasty movies such as the *Texas Chainsaw Massacre* also keep locals on edge. That being said, there are also trigger-happy individuals who don't want you anywhere near their property. That's why PSL Ranch has *no tresspassing* signs posted all around our ranch's boundary... that and because Cassy likes shooting at strangers whenever she gets the chance.

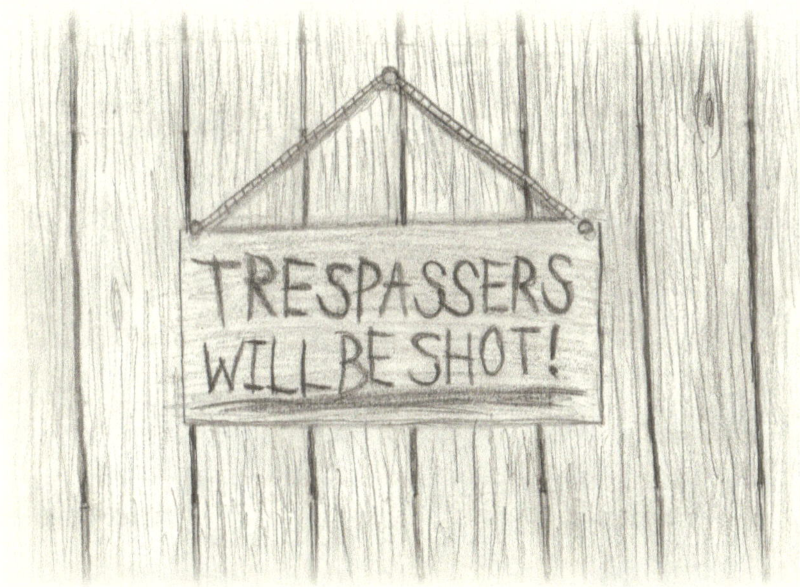

During one GTCA camper outing in the middle of hunting season, a group of campers were running into a local rancher's property, ringing his cow bell, and running back to PSL Ranch. They thought this act of passive aggression was fun, as when the cows heard the bell they would all come running for hay. The old rancher who owned the property, Bo Jingles, was getting mighty irritated as the cattle were becoming aggressive without their hay! It seems one of PSL's ranch hands (probably Cookie) had told a campfire story about how other campers did this as a game and they wanted to share in this false tradition. What happened next was witnessed by Funny Boy and reported to the Menard County sheriff's department in the following statement:

"I was out picking milk thistles for Cookie's soup when I heard the faint sound of Bo Jingle's cowbell over and over. I thought, crap, the campers must have thought the story I told… I mean that Cookie told them was true! I went running toward them as fast as I could when I heard a single shot from Bo's .375 H&H! Then all I heard was screaming and a bunch of campers running as fast as they could back to the ranch house. I counted them as they ran by; one, two, three… ten, eleven. My stomach sank as I knew there were 12 in all!

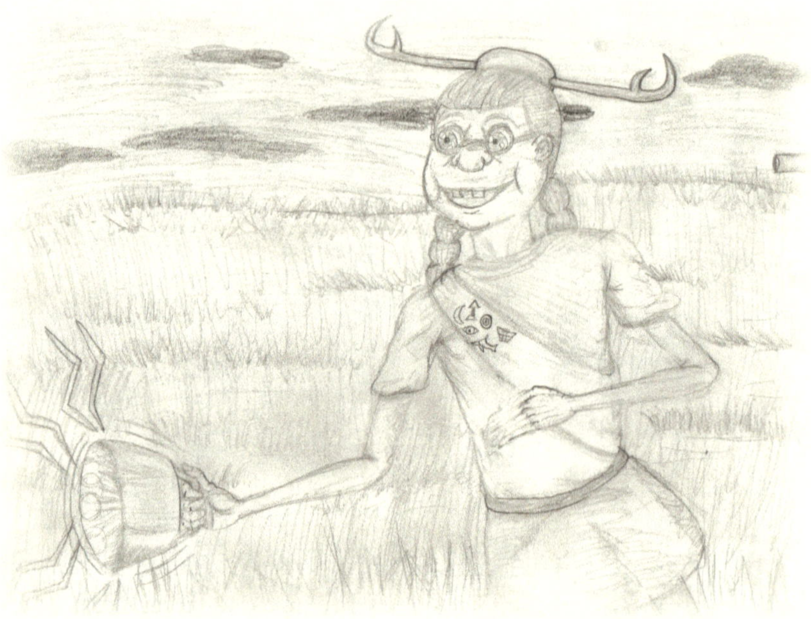

Apparently, Sally was at the end of the line and the other campers chided her to go and ring the bell for the last time. She did and it was the last time she ever would!

Menard County Sheriff Buck Mueller, ruled the incident illegal trespassing and PSL Ranch not liable for the following reasons:

1. It was clearly trespassing.
2. Old Bo is an excellent shot, especially with his elephant gun.
3. Cookie and Funny Boy blamed each other, and determination of guilt could not be established.

PSL Ranch administrators felt mighty awful about the clean shot on Sally's head, so to prevent future incidents as well as to maintain good relations with old Bo, we now provide some simple facts about trespassing laws for new guests visiting our pristine little piece of Texas:

- It is not lawful to shoot someone in Texas who is merely trespassing.
- It is lawful in Texas to display your firearm to create apprehension that you will use deadly force if necessary (Castle Doctrine).
- A property owner has no legal responsibility to run away from a situation where he or she feels threatened.
- It is legal to shoot to kill in Texas if you feel your property is threatened.

Well it was obvious to all that old Bo felt his property was threatened as his cattle were starting to tear up his barn due to the campers trespassing pranks.

Conclusion: Don't Trespass!

Incident #27

Flashflood: Why Do You Think the Cabin's on Stilts?

Vanishing of a GTCA Camper

You may have heard the old saying, "When it rains, it pours." This saying doesn't reflect actual weather patterns, but rather, refers to non-weather related events, so it has no bearing on this incident.

What does have a direct relationship with a vanishing GTCA camper was a sudden flashflood that occurred when there was only a 20 percent chance of rain. Yes, flashfloods can come out of nowhere and sometimes they last for hours and vanish as quickly as they started. The end-result can be a torrent of water rushing over the flatlands to the wash—our lowest point on the property. The water can be four to eight inches deep and may move quickly over the banks and downstream to the San Saba River. This is why the ranch house is nestled on a pier and beam foundation three feet above the ground; as well as an unintentional design deviation with a very positive result!

On one fateful late spring afternoon, several GTCA campers were watching large storm clouds approach from the West. They were public school Northerners who were taught to believe everything the government tells you to, including those that work for the National Weather Service. On their way to PSL Ranch earlier in the day, it was reported there was a 20 percent chance of light rain, so as far as the campers were concerned, the worst that could happen is they would get a little wet. Once at PSL Ranch the campers saw a flock of turkeys running around just a few hundred yards from the ranch house.

110

They decided to go chase them and see if they could catch one for Cookie's evening meal as they were tired of possum and grits; then the rain began to fall. Unfortunately for one GTCA camper named Sally, it was a little more than she bargained for. What happened next was witnessed by Shari Running Wild who was hugging her favorite live oak high above the ground:

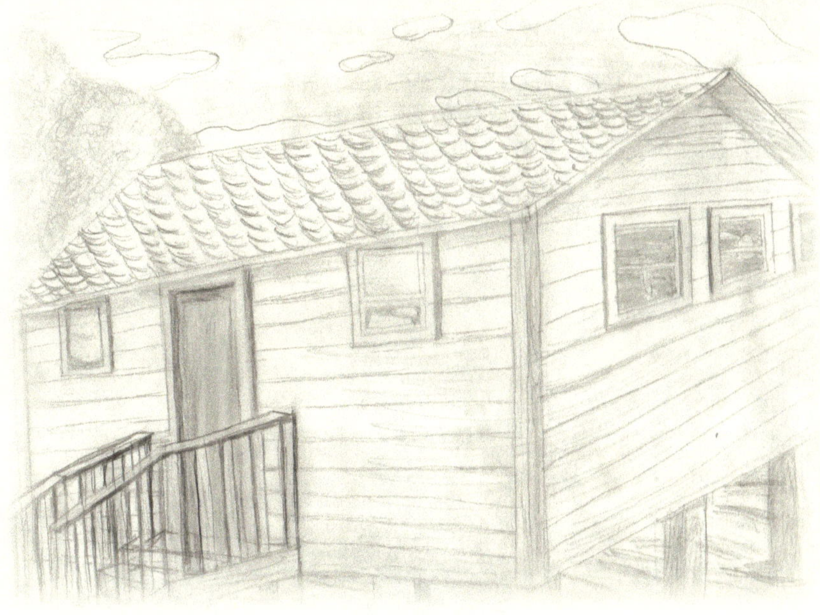

"Rain come hard. Campers run with turkey. Sally wash away."

What the Campers didn't realize is that a heavy rain storm dumped inches of rain just East of PSL Ranch before heading West and soaking the campgrounds. Sally, being distracted while she tried to catch a turkey, didn't notice the water level rising, and by the time she did it was already six inches deep and rushing over the banks of Lake Rohret (previously the wash). As she tried to run back to the ranch house, she was knocked over by the swiftly flowing water and carried downstream never to be seen again!

Menard County Sheriff Buck Mueller ruled the incident death by gully washer, and that PSL Ranch was not liable for the following reasons:

1. It was obviously a case of poor weather forecasting by the National Weather Service.
2. It wasn't turkey season.
3. God was calling Sally home, and because she couldn't be found, she must have made it.

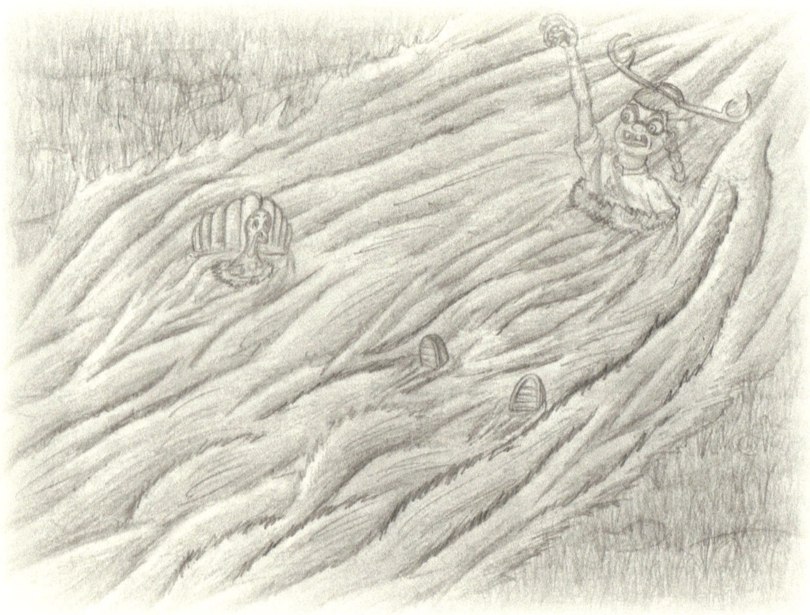

Because Shari Running Wild was stuck up a tree for several hours before the water abated, and GTCA camp coordinators did not take roll to see who made it back, it was hours before anyone realized Sally was missing. We at PSL Ranch take no responsibility for this unfortunate incident; all the same, we now take painstaking efforts to educate visitors on the dangers associated with a flashflood by providing some interesting facts:

- Except for heat-related fatalities, more deaths occur from flooding than any other hazard.
- Most people fail to realize the power of water; six inches of fast-moving flood water can knock you off your feet.
- The national thirty-year average for flood deaths in the United States is 127.
- Most victims are male (no one told Sally!).
- Flood deaths affect all age groups.
- Most flashfloods are caused by slow moving thunderstorms.
- Flashfloods can develop within minutes or hours depending on the intensity and duration of the rain, the topography, soil conditions, and ground cover.

Of course, knowing any of these facts would not have saved Sally, but they are interesting!

Conclusion: Don't chase the turkeys!

<h1 style="text-align:center">Incident #28</h1>

<h1 style="text-align:center">Death by Archery or Robin
Hood She Ain't!</h1>

Archery Accident Causing the Death of a GTCA Camper

Archery is a sport that predates written history; requiring balance, strength, and skills developed through lots of practice. Archery is also a sport that has been glamorized in movies and animated features showing impossible shots and even horse-play that always seems to end well for the main characters (except Errol Flynn in his role as Custer). PSL Ranch provides an excellent archery range for our visitors to practice their sport if they already know how to use a bow and arrow, or to train young eager campers in the art of hitting the target at which they are aiming. PSL Ranch's archery instructor is no other than our resident inju —… 2.4 percent Native American, Shari Running Wild. Whatever tribe she hailed from knew how to shoot the eyes out of a rattlesnake, and that skill was passed down to her!

On one cool spring day (less than 100 degrees), Shari Running Wild was instructing a group of young campers in the art of using an authentic, ancient Indian compound bow. What happened next is detailed in the following testimonial provided to the Menard County sheriff's department by Dr. S who witnessed everything:

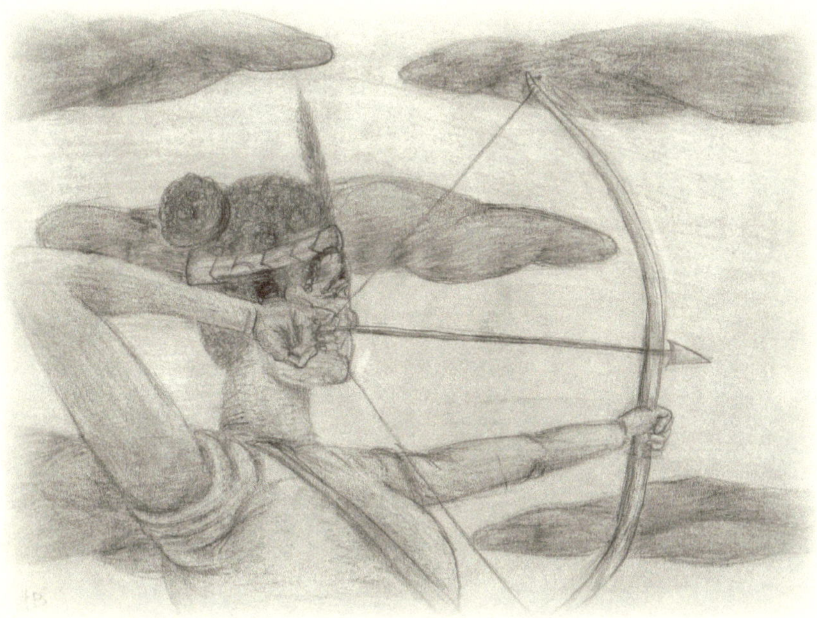

"It was about noon as the Sun was directly overhead when I began watching Shari Running Wild instruct the campers. I should be the lead instructor as it was I who put an arrow in the back of another from thirty yards, not Running Wild, and it was I who made the University of Chicago's archery team, and it was I who had to show Running Wild how to fix her sights on her compound bow, and it is me who is better at instructing students. But nooo, Slim always liked Running Wild better and gives her all the good jobs! I never get to…"

Sheriff Mueller interrupted, "Dr. S, please get to the point!"

Dr. S continued, "Oh, sorry. Anyway, while Running Wild was showing one student how to nock her arrow, another student named Sally was messing around and not listening. She was pretending to be the Arrow or some other comic book character when all of a sudden she aimed directly up and let her arrow loose right into the Sun. No one could see where it was going to land as it was too bright, but we all found out a moment later when it came straight down entering the top of her head and piercing her body lengthwise. I have no idea why Running Wild had them all using hunting points!"

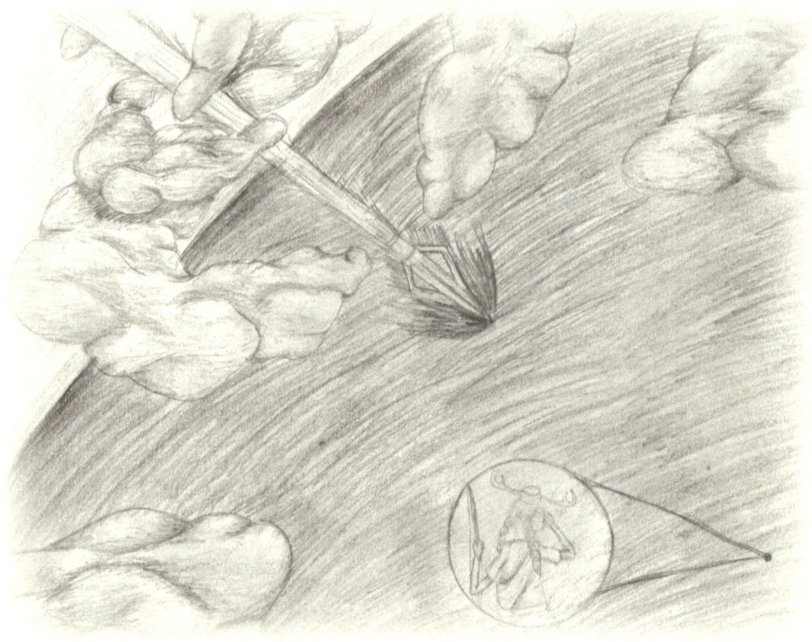

Well it was instant death for the GTCA camper, Sally, who unwittingly hit her first target with her first shot! Although stunned, the other students completed their training as there was nothing they could do about Sally anyway.

Menard County Sheriff, Buck Mueller, ruled the incident unintentional suicide and that PSL Ranch was not liable for the following reasons:

1. Sally should have been listening to her instructor and not messing around.
2. It wasn't human season yet in Texas.
3. Robin Hood she wasn't!

Although fifteen or twenty previous campers were hit by stray arrows in the past, this was the first fatality from archery on PSL Ranch. To prevent future unintentional suicide by arrow, Slim appointed Dr. S as the new instructor and provides a few facts about archery to newcomers at the ranch.

- There are approximately 3,900 injuries annually due to archery-related accidents associated with over 6.8 million archers.
- In the United States, there have been multiple deaths from archery accidents and over twenty murders using the bow and arrow.
- Sally is the first recorded suicide by bow and arrow.

These statistics clearly show how safe archery is and that future visitors to PSL Ranch should feel at ease with this sport.

Conclusion: Don't aim at the Sun!

Dehydration Is Only Good for Fruit and Meat

Death of a GTCA Camper Due to Lack of Water

While hiking in a hot, dry climate, it is essential that hikers remain hydrated by drinking lots of water. This includes packing enough water for your trip with a reserve supply in case you misjudge. Because PSL Ranch is in a semi-arid location without a good source of clean water on remote areas of the property, ranch hands stress the need to carry a backpack or camel back whenever hiking or working beyond sight of the ranch house. Hiking is a safe sport and provides excellent exercise for everyone when precautions are taken.

On a hot mid-August day just after breakfast, a group of GTCA campers decided to take a long hike around the ranch's perimeter. This long hike would take them the rest of the afternoon and long into the evening, so they all packed four quarts of water, snacks consisting of energy bars, and a bottle or two of electrolyte water. These campers were eager to go and didn't mind the extra ten pounds of supplies—except for one, Sally. She immediately began complaining of the extra weight and whined the first thirty minutes of the trip. What happened later in the hike was witnessed by Cookie who happened to be at her still cooking up some good mash:

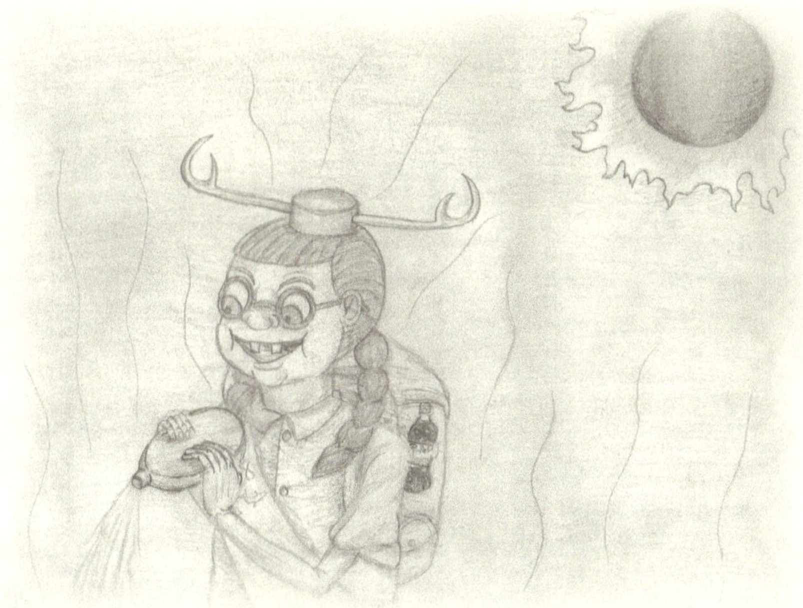

"Being of good German stock, I routinely hump forty gallons of water to my still… I means, my scientific experiment. I just finished a couple of pints of my medicinal brew when I hurd them pesky campers clompin' down the West side of the wash scarin' every critter a mile around! I saws one, I thinks it was Sally, mumbling to herself and walking kinda funny, stumblin' and all. I went up to the GTCA counselor and asked, 'What's up with the funny lookin' one?' She said that it was just Sally and that she always acts weird and can't keep up, so I thoughts no more of it. Later, on my way back to the ranch house, I found a shriveled-up girl that looked like she slept the night in Slim's smokehouse. It was Sally all right, dead as a fish outta water!"

Apparently, Sally was tired of carrying her water and dumped it before they were halfway through their hike. She also replaced her energy bars with a couple of bags of sea salt potato chips, which helped to dehydrate her and hasten her demise.

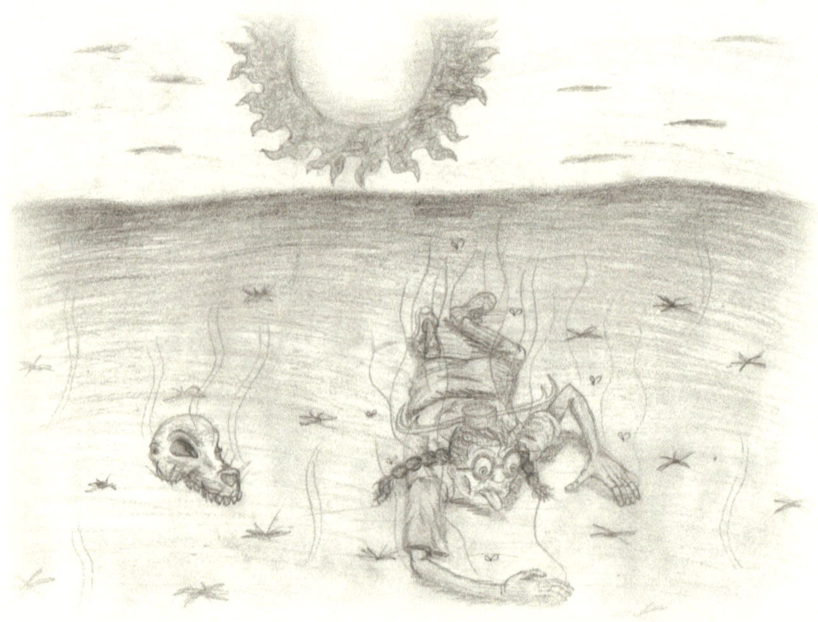

Menard County Sheriff, Buck Mueller, ruled the incident a fatal case of laziness and that PSL Ranch was not liable for the following reasons:

1. The campers were all briefed about the dangers of dehydration prior to their hike.
2. Cookie correctly inquired as to the health of the funny looking one.
3. It was clearly the GTCA counselor's fault as she was leading the hike!

This incident was obviously avoidable but was definitely not the fault of PSL Ranch! To decrease the likelihood of similar incidents like this one, PSL administrators now provide some facts about dehydration to our guests such as the following common symptoms:

- Increased thirst
- Dry mouth
- Tiredness or sleepiness
- Urine is low volume and more yellowish than normal
- Headache
- Dry skin
- Dizziness

Another interesting fact is that dehydration results in approximately 200,000 hospitalizations and three hundred deaths per year.

Conclusion: Don't dump your water!

If You ain't Trained with a Gun, Don't Use It!

Accidental Shooting Death of a GTCA Camper

One Texas trait you may have become aware of while reading this educational treatise on conservation and safety is that Texans like their guns. Pistols, rifles, shotguns, black powder, antique, and customized sidearms are all available to provide recreation and security for the populous of this wonderful state. It should be no surprise that many of the summer youth camps in Texas provide recreational target shooting as one of their activities. Because guns are numerous, even a way of life for some Texans. These youth camps play an important role in properly training future hunters and recreational marksmen.

PSL Ranch also provides a shooting range for our campers and guests who want to try their luck hitting the zombie targets Funny Boy placed downrange. GTCA campers are especially interested in our shooting courses as most are from liberal states and have never touched, or even seen, a real gun.

PSL's ranch hands are adamant about safety all the time, but even more so when it comes to our gun course. So when it came time to select an instructor, Slim chose the most experienced and qualified on the ranch, Cassy. Cassy never misses what she shoots at and is considered an expert with every weapon owned by PSL Ranch. Furthermore, Cassy has never had an accident, or she has always been acquitted by Menard County judges every time there was one.

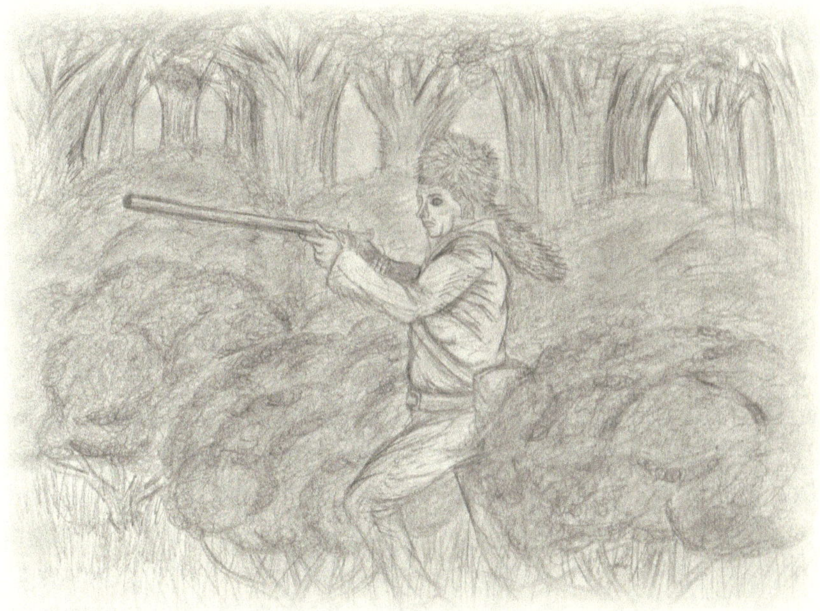

On one clear summer morning, a group of twelve-year-old GTCA campers excitedly ran to the gun range to try their hand at zombie killing. They were first lined up and given the mandatory safety briefing by Slim who emphasized that they should listen to, and comply with, whatever Cassy said. Slim was a little worried (he always is) as several of the campers were not paying attention and were horsing around. What happened next was witnessed by Dr. S and relayed to the Menard County sheriff's department.

"I was out and about trying to find Shari Running Wild who was supposed to be cleaning the kitchen. She always finds a way to shirk her duties, and I end up getting stuck with whatever she decides she doesn't want to do! If I forget to do something, I get scolded, but Slim and Cassy let her get away with everything! In fact,… sorry, I'll get to the point. I saw Slim give his lackluster safety briefing, and as usual, he was nervous; talking too fast and leaving out important details like, "Don't load your weapons until you are told to do so." Then Cassy began passing out the guns. Johnny got the Chinese SKS, a sweet semi-auto assault rifle; Judy got the .50 Cal. black powder long gun with a range of eight hundred yards; Billy and Marsha got the .38 and .45 pistols; Sally got the twelve gauge—which was more than she could handle; Bernie got the 1936 French Mas, which can't hit anything, and Harold got the rat gun. Harold was pissed! He wanted Slim's sidearm, an 1851 Navy .36 cal, but Slim gives that gun to no one! As a rule, everyone leaves their gun on the table except for the one shooting, but Harold went up and grabbed the rat gun out of turn. Cassy then said, "Drop di gun pickney! Yu waa kill sumdoy?" Harold just looked at her puzzled and began playing with it. It all went downhill from there! Harold pulled the trigger and nearly shot Judy. Judy swung around and fired off her .50 Cal. knocking her ten feet back. Startled, Billy, who was up at the table, started shooting his 1911 .45 in every direction until it was empty. Then Marsha, Johnny, Bernie, and Harold continued shooting until their weapons were empty. Once the whole event was over, and I emerged from behind the barn, I remembered the only gun I didn't hear was the pump 12 gauge. That's when I realized the only one hit in the high-noon event, was Sally."

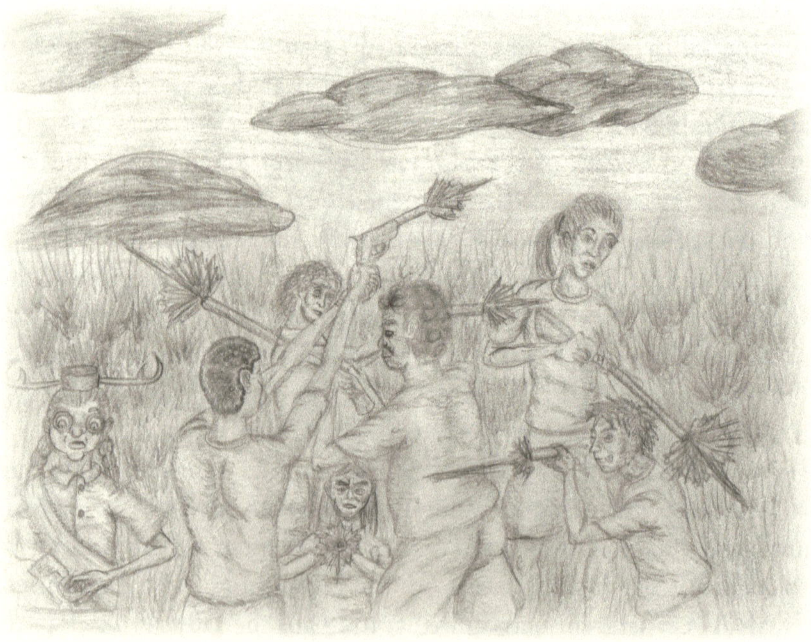

Apparently, with over thirty-nine bullets flying in every direction, it was one from the rat gun that hit Sally in the temple, killing her instantly.

Menard County Sheriff, Buck Mueller, ruled the incident an intentional homicide, and that PSL Ranch was not liable for the following reasons:

1. Cassy recognized the danger and clearly told Harold to put the gun down.
2. Everyone else was able to miss Sally, so Harold could have missed as well if he wanted to.
3. The bullet that killed Sally was from Harold's gun!

Sheriff Mueller took the findings from his fifteen-minute investigation to the Menard District Attorney, Ms. T, who after a brief review and a pint of Cookie's aged moonshine, recommended that Harold be charged with murder as an adult. Adding, "If he's old enough to use the gun, he's old enough to suffer the consequences!" Menard County's District Judge, Rob Hangman, immediately arranged for a jury of twelve, which happened to be those attending his family reunion and who quickly found Harold guilty. The death sentence was then announced and local carpenters began building the gallows.

It was later learned that anyone under the age of 18 in the State of Texas is considered a minor and Judge Hangman was overruled. Harold is now undergoing therapy, but spends most of his time in the fetal position muttering, "I thought she was a rat!" Judge Hangman used the gallows for a community bonfire.

PSL Ranch administrators were nervous, but relieved that the Ranch was cleared of all wrongdoing. To ensure an incident like this one never happens again, Slim was replaced by Dr. S as the safety briefer. We also provide a few gun-related facts for those visiting our little piece of heaven to make everyone safer during our shooting course:

- Always keep the muzzle pointed in a safe direction, not at Sally.

- Firearms should remain unloaded when not in use.
- Don't trust your gun's safety.
- Know your target and what's behind it.
- Use the correct ammunition.
- Receive lessons from an English speaker, not a Patois speaker.
- If your gun fails to fire, be very cautious.
- Always wear eye and ear protection.
- Be sure the barrel is clear of obstructions.
- Don't alter or modify your gun unless it's by a licensed gunsmith.
- Have guns serviced regularly.
- Know how to handle your firearm.

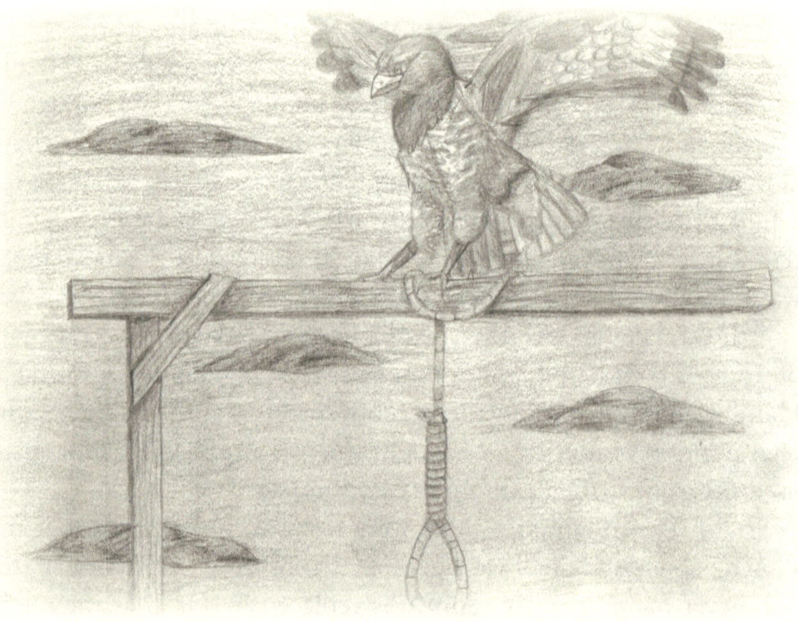

Conclusion: Don't play with guns!

INCIDENT #31

Heatstroke: The Microwave Effect!

Death of a GTCA Camper Due to Heatstroke

The summer sun in Texas can be brutal, reaching high temperatures of 100–110 degrees Fahrenheit over extended periods. The hottest temperature recorded in Texas was 120 degrees Fahrenheit in Seymour, a town about halfway between Menard and Dallas. Working and living in severe heat has become a way of life for most Texans, but many cases of heat related illnesses still occur annually.

Heatstroke, heat exhaustion, and other heat-related illnesses can be prevented if their symptoms are recognized in time. Although dehydration is a common factor, it should be noted that even well-hydrated individuals can succumb to heat-related illnesses. When working or hiking in extremely warm temperatures, you should restrict activities to prevent overheating which includes resting in shaded or air-conditioned locations when possible.

On a mid-August afternoon, a group of GTCA campers from Alaska decided to travel to the far South region of PSL Ranch to observe a flock of turkeys that inhabit the area. To prevent dehydration, like incident #29, Slim made sure each camper drank twenty ounces of water in his presence and that each camper had two liters of extra water in his or her packs. Furthermore, he briefed the GTCA counselor of what can happen if the campers didn't have enough water for the trip.

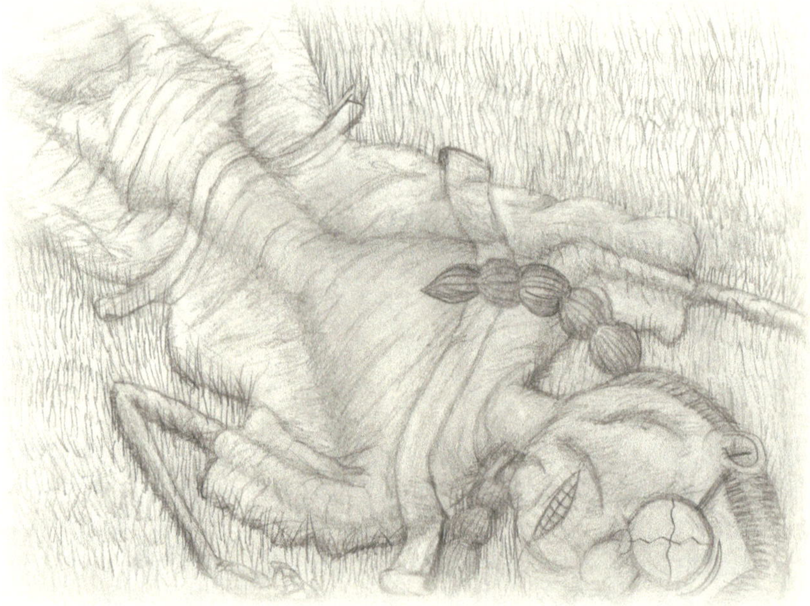

The expedition then left and hurried across the approved wash-trail, making its way through thick brush, cactus, and mesquite trees. The going was rough, and each camper was sweating profusely, drinking plenty of water along the way. Because they were behind schedule, the campers continued without breaks for most of the afternoon and several became nauseated and dizzy, particularly one camper named Sally. What happened next was witnessed by Shari Running Wild who was searching for turkey feathers for a ceremonial headdress she was going to use during an upcoming rain dance:

"Sally turn red. Sally walk in circle. Sally drop dead."

Apparently, Sally had not acclimated to the hot Texas sun, and although she was well hydrated, the intense hiking raised her body temperature to 105 degrees causing disorientation, nausea, and redness before expiring. Her symptoms were not immediately recognized as most campers are nauseous following Cookie's meals and the GTCA counselor stated Sally was always a little dizzy!

Menard County Sheriff, Buck Mueller, ruled the incident a case of baked-brain syndrome, and that PSL Ranch was not liable for the following reasons:

1. PSL Ranch does not control the weather unless you're talking about Shari Running Wild's ability to summon rain.
2. The GTCA counselor should have noticed something was wrong.
3. Who hikes for hours to look at turkeys?

Relieved at being exonerated, PSL Ranch still feels the need to better explain heat-related illnesses to prevent future incidents of this type. The following facts are therefore provided to all PSL Ranch visitors.

Symptoms of heat-related illnesses:

- Severe and throbbing headache
- Dizziness and light-headedness (more than usual if your name is Sally)
- Lack of sweating despite the heat—even if hydrated
- Red, hot, and dry skin
- Muscle weakness and cramps
- Nausea and vomiting (may be due to Cookie's meals, but don't take a chance)
- Rapid heartbeat
- Rapid, shallow breathing
- Confusion, disorientation, or staggering
- Seizures
- Body temperature of 104 degrees or greater
- Unconsciousness

If you suspect a camper has heatstroke, call 911 or transport the victim to a hospital immediately; a delay in seeking medical help can be fatal. While waiting for help, which may take a while at PSL Ranch, move the person to air-conditioning or a shady area and remove unnecessary clothing. Other ways to cooldown a suspected heatstroke victim include:

- Wet their clothes or skin and fan air over them
- If available, apply ice packs to the victim's armpits, groin, neck, and back
- Immerse the victim in a tub of cool water or a shower

We hope these facts can help visitors to our paradise quickly identify symptoms of overheating. If you or another hiker exhibit one or more of these symptoms, stop to rest, hydrate, and cooldown.

Conclusion: Don't hike after eating one of Cookies' famous meals!

The Brown Recluse, Black Widow, and Other Nasty Spiders

Death of a GTCA Camper Due to Poisonous Spider Bites

Like most places in the United States, Texas has its share of poisonous spiders lurking in trees, brush piles, and even in the kitchen pantry. They are not more numerous on PSL Ranch than any other location, but visitors should be alerted to the types of spiders and symptoms of a spider bite so it can be treated accordingly. No, spiders do not team up with snakes to attack campers like feral hogs and axis deer do, but all the same, several types of spiders can live in near proximity, and like everything else on PSL Ranch, can hurt you if accidently provoked!

The two most common poisonous spiders on PSL Ranch are the *Latrodectus mactans* (Southern Black Widow) and the *Loxosceles reclusa* (Brown Recluse). Both are capable of inflicting nasty bites that have very different effects on their victims. Cassy's favorite is the Southern Black Widow due to the female's habit of killing and sucking the blood out of a male spider after breeding. In contrast, Cassy thinks the Brown Recluse is boring as it won't actually kill a human, but rather, just causes flesh to rot and fall off.

On one chilly spring morning on PSL Ranch, a group of Oregon-based GTCA campers left their encampment to hunt for some dry firewood for a campfire. None of the campers wanted to eat Cookie's possum-tail and egg omelets that morning and the last of the store-bought cereal was gone, so they stole a can of Slim's spam and decided to cook it over a fire.

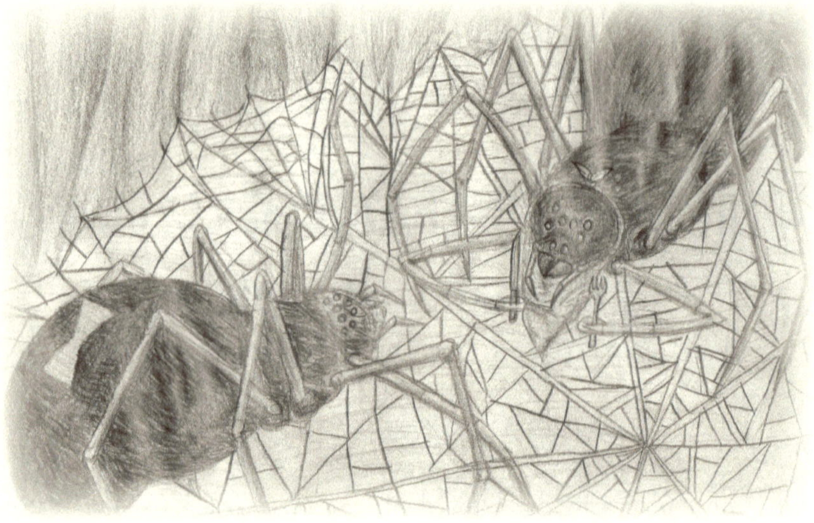

As they combed the East bank of Lake Rohret, they noticed a large pile of brush containing a lot of dead live oak branches. They immediately began to reach into the pile to pull out small branches for their fire. One camper, named Salli (pronounced Sally—with an *I*), was the ringleader and was especially aggressive in obtaining wood. What happened next was witnessed by Cassy who saw them steal Slim's spam and followed them to see what was going on. The following eyewitness account was provided to the Menard Sheriff's department:

"Mi si dem pickney teef Slim spam, so mi tek a stick to lik dem. Mi faala di pickney dem to an ole wood pile. Den, all of a sudden, Sally wid an *I* scream an run le. Di res a di pickney faala are, so mi nevah afta to lik dem."

English Translation: I saw some children steal Slim's spam, so I grabbed a stick to whack them with and followed them to an old wood pile. Sally-with-an-I screamed and they all ran away so I didn't get to whack them!

About twenty minutes later, the ornery group of campers returned to camp, and Sally with an *I* was holding her wrist. She was also nauseated, had muscle cramps, was dizzy, and had a rapid pulse. Slim knew the symptoms; it was heatstroke! Dr. S reminded Slim that it was only 53 degrees outside, so the probability of heatstroke was one in a thousand. Funny Boy began to disagree with Dr. S because he couldn't verify her information on the Internet, therefore, it wasn't true. Cookie got into the fray and started yelling between gulps of beer, "What the hell is wrong with my possum omelets!" Cassy thought it might be a bite of some kind but was having too much fun whacking the campers with a stick to intervene. Suddenly, Shari Running Wild yelled, "Girl dead."

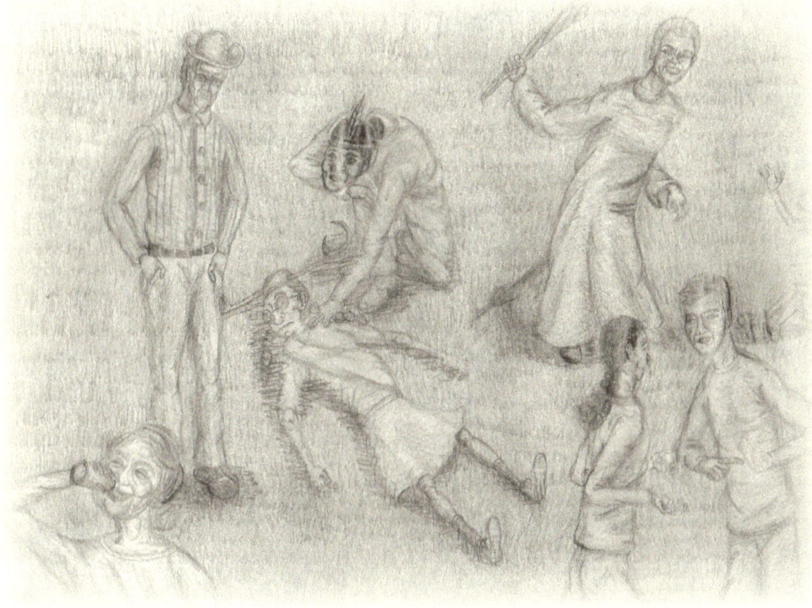

Menard County Sheriff, Buck Mueller, ruled the incident death by Arachnid, and that PSL Ranch was not liable for the following reasons:

1. Sally with an *I* was a thief.
2. Spiders, like humans in Menard County, Texas, are allowed to protect their property using deadly force.
3. Cookie's possum omelets are good eatin'!

Apparently, the venom reached Sally with an *I*'s nervous system before medical help could be obtained. All of the PSL Ranch hands felt bad about the incident except Slim who was still irritated that his last can of spam had been pinched. All the same, Slim now provides the following facts about the two most numerous poisonous spiders on the property to help prevent future cases of death by Arachnid.

Southern Black Widow Spider facts:

- Severe pain is usually felt immediately at the location of the bite.
- Localized or generalized severe muscle cramps, abdominal pain, weakness, and tremors follow, usually in about twenty to sixty minutes.
- In severe cases, nausea, vomiting, fainting, dizziness, chest pain, and respiratory difficulties occur.
- Children and old folks are more seriously affected, especially those named Sally with an *I*.
- In some cases, abdominal pain may mimic such conditions as appendicitis or gallbladder problems.
- Chest pain may be mistaken for a heart attack.
- Blood pressure and heart rate may be elevated.
- Many of the symptoms also mimic heatstroke—but if it's cold, it's probably only one in a thousand chance of being heatstroke.
- Southern Black Widow Spiders are often found in concealed areas such as brush piles and enclosed areas.
- Rarely do bites result in death.
- Most medical facilities do not have the ability to provide assistance—so don't get bit.
- Mostly found in the Southern states like Texas.

Brown Recluse Spider facts:

- Unlike the Southern Black Widow Spider, Brown Recluse bites don't hurt, and you may not even know you were bitten.
- Symptoms may not appear for several hours, at which time, you may begin experiencing stinging or a burning sensation at the bite location.
- A unique pattern of discoloration will develop around the bite, which may turn deep purple or blue surrounded by a whitish ring and a large red area.
- A nasty ulcer may develop and persist for several weeks.
- Other symptoms include fever, nausea, rash, chills, itching, sweating, and rotting body parts (most of the time, the symptoms are not that bad).
- If bitten, wash wound area with soap, elevate, and apply an ice pack, then get your ass to the hospital.

The following website provides detailed descriptions of these two spiders as well as other spiders common to PSL Ranch: http://www.termite.com/spider-identification.html. PSL Ranch also provides visitors with a spider identification guide as there is no Internet on the ranch.

Conclusion: Don't steal Slim's spam!

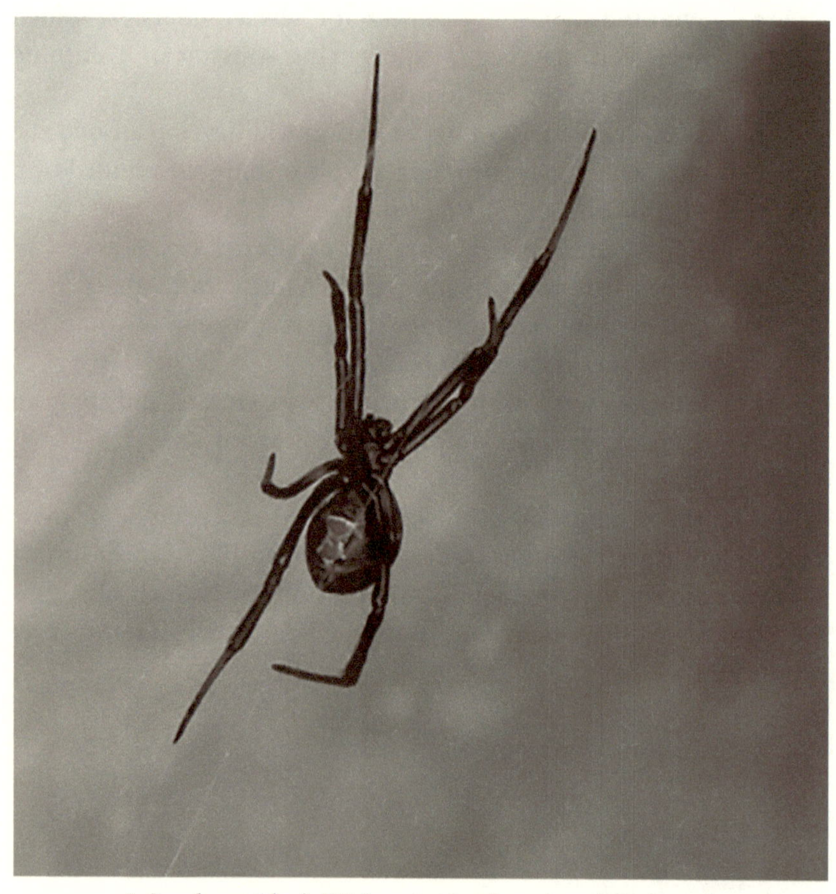

A Southern Black Widow Spider found on PSL Ranch

Lyme Disease: The Dreaded Tick or Government Conspiracy?

Contraction of Lyme Disease by a GTCA Camper

Lyme disease is named after the location of its first breakout, Lyme, Connecticut, which happens to be across from a US Government biosafety level three laboratory located on Plum Island. Authorities at Plum Island deny that they are the cause of the dreaded weaponized disease as they destroy every animal on the island following research, but it should be noted that birds fly between the island and the mainland unencumbered; and ticks, which spread Lyme disease, stick to birds. Lyme disease can now be found across the United States and on every continent except Antarctica. Those bitten by an infected tick may go decades without knowing that their chronic ailments are due to Lyme disease, all the time making their lives miserable and eventually causing or contributing to their death.

In his book *Lab 257*, Michael C. Carroll, makes the case that the Plum Island animal disease center was the cause for an infectious Lyme outbreak in 1975. Many conspiracy theorists, including Slim, now believe that the Plum Island facility was used for bioweapon research following WWII through the end of the Cold War. This whacky conspiracy was provided some credibility when the US Government decided to build a twenty-two-thousand-square foot research center in San Antonio, Texas, to research biotech weapons including Lyme disease.[6]

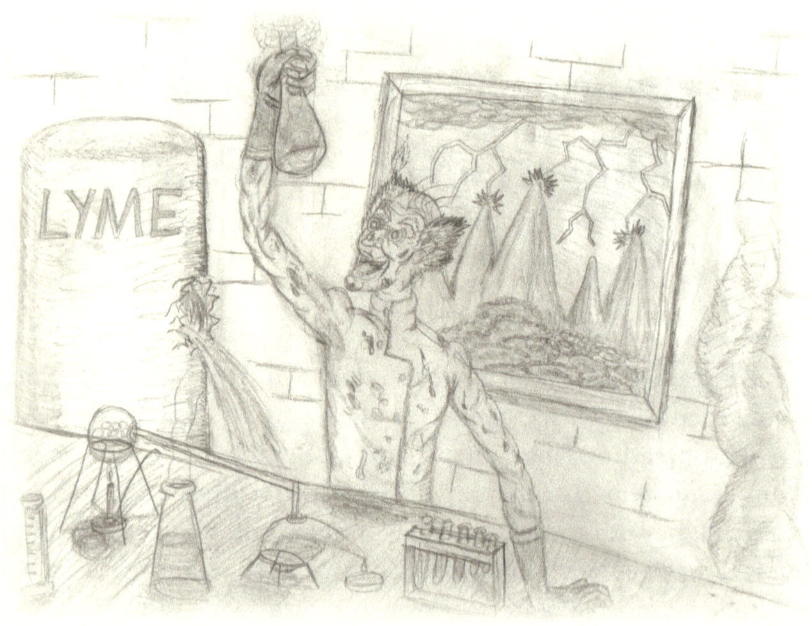

Why are PSL Ranch hands concerned with Lyme disease? Because everywhere there are deer there are ticks, and the ticks that like deer may be infected with Lyme disease. In fact, there are areas where Lyme disease is so prevalent that it is illegal to skin a deer outside of the county in which it was shot to help prevent the spread of the disease. Although most of the ranch hands at PSL Ranch exhibit symptoms, such as tiredness, soreness, and forgetfulness, they are just lazy for the most part and aren't infected. Unfortunately for one GTCA camper from Connecticut, named Sally, that would not be the case.

Recently, around the time of the 2016 elections, Sally returned to Connecticut following a camping holiday at PSL Ranch with her GTCA troop. Sally became ill shortly after returning home with

---

6. http://www.msnbc.msn.com/id/10039154/.

symptoms that included memory loss, cognitive confusion, and vision problems. On November 5, 2016, she mistakenly put on her little brothers *Vote Trump* T-shirt, and in a cognitively-confused state, wondered into a group of peace-loving progressives who proceeded to stone her to death after they spit on her and called her names. Connecticut's district attorney saw nothing wrong with these actions, but decided to request a statement from PSL Ranch hands after they discovered Sally had become infected with Lyme disease; after all, progressives like to sue!

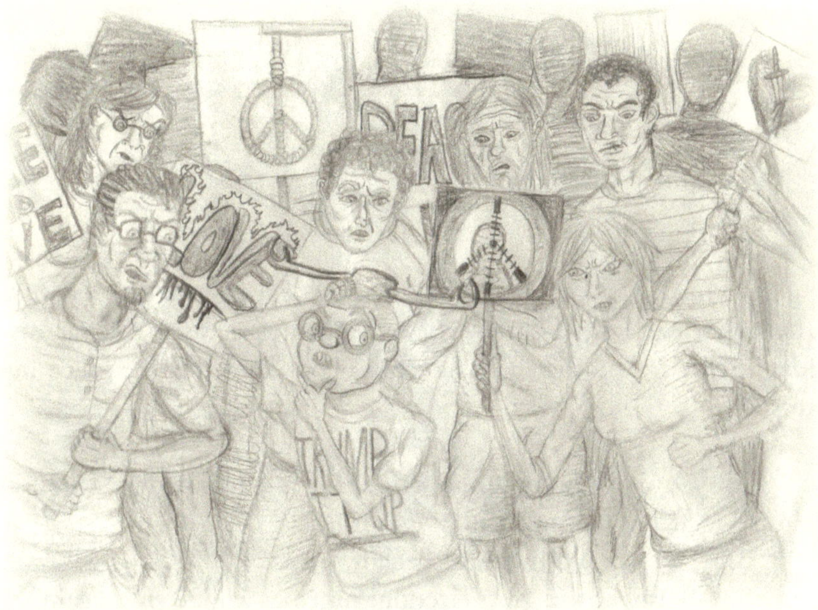

The following testimonial was provided to the Menard County sheriff's department by Cookie, who kind of remembered the incident:

"I was cleaning the copper tubing used on still number four because sumthin' was pluggin' it up. When I saw them silly lookin' campin' girls returnin' from the deer feeder where they was watchin' the deer. I told 'em to check for ticks, and they all laughed pointing at Sally sayin' she had a tick. I thoughts nothin' of it as she was always jerkin', and I thoughts that's what they meant."

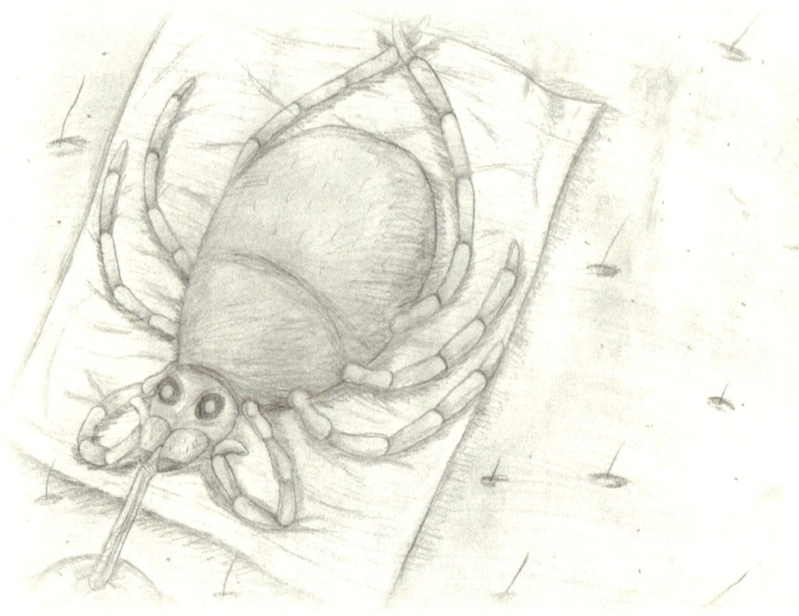

Menard County Sheriff, Buck Mueller—wearing a *Make America Great Again* T-shirt—ruled the incident a case of liberal misidentification, and that PSL Ranch was not liable for the following reasons:

1. Connecticut has more cases of Lyme disease than Texas, so suck it Connecticut.
2. Cookie told them to check for ticks.
3. Wasn't that a great election! America will be *great* again!

Not knowing exactly what Sheriff Mueller's comments meant, PSL Ranch administrators welcomed the exoneration. They also decided to provide some basic facts about deer ticks, Lyme disease, and prevention:

1. Lyme disease is a worldwide infectious disease and has been reported in all fifty states.
2. Lyme disease is transmitted through a bite from an infected deer tick.

3. Deer ticks are the size of a poppy seed and can leave an undetectable bite.
4. A bull's-eye rash may develop around the bite.
5. Some victims develop flu-like symptoms a week or so after becoming infected; however, many people are asymptomatic and may develop Lyme symptoms months, years, or decades later.
6. Symptoms include fatigue, neck pain, jaw pain, muscle pain, joint pain, swollen glands, memory loss, confusion, vision problems, digestive problems, headaches, fainting, and sometimes death.
7. Lyme disease is growing at epidemic proportions in the United States. In 2013, the CDC estimated three hundred thousand new cases annually up from thirty thousand in 2009.
8. If you suspect you have Lyme, contact a Lyme literate medical Doctor (LLMD).
9. You can only get Lyme disease from a tick bite and not all ticks carry Lyme disease.
10. In most cases, it takes thirty to forty-eight hours for an infected tick to transmit Lyme disease after it attaches itself to you.
11. Most cases of Lyme disease can be treated and cured with antibiotics.
12. Take the following precautions to prevent Lyme disease:
    - If you're going outdoors in a grassy or wooded area, wear light-colored long-sleeved shirts and long pants to make ticks easier to spot.
    - Spray clothing with permethrin repellent.
    - Spray DEET directly on your skin.
    - Following outdoor activities, check for ticks all over your body.
    - Wash all clothing.
    - Taking a bath with one-fourth to one-half cup of household bleach will cause an undetected attached tick to *blackout*.

We hope these facts help calm any fears of possible Lyme infection at PSL Ranch, and we hope to see you as a guest in the near future!

Conclusion: Don't get ticked!

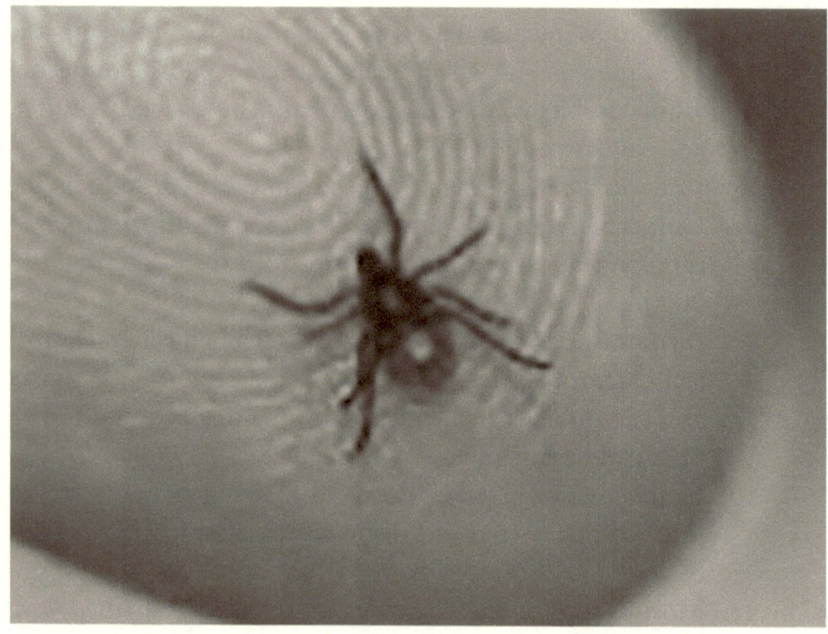

Deer Ticks are extremely small and hard to see

Incident #34

Openly Supporting Gun Control

Another Appalling Suicide by a GTCA Camper

If there's one topic that stirs emotions in Texas, it's gun laws, specifically gun control. It's not that Texans want anyone to be able to easily purchase a fully equipped M1 Abrahams tank or a used Trident Missile complete with launch silo—because we don't.[7] It's just that those timid souls up North who are unwilling to defend themselves think that criminals are victims and not responsible for their own actions. They preach that everyone should think as they do and accept fate as it comes. Texans are in the business of creating their own destiny, and we tempt fate daily. Apparently, progressives believe every crime is a direct result of a gun, not the user.

In contrast the descendants of central Texas settlers, and those that have arrived since, take a slightly different approach to criminals and rogue government actions. Like most Texans; White, Black, Hispanic, Native American, or (fill in your favorite race, color, sexual preference, gender identification, or religion here—we don't judge) ___________________________, we believe it's our duty to accept responsibility for our own actions. Why the long preamble to incident #34? This background information is necessary to fully understand what happened to Sally at her candidate's rally in San Angelo, Texas, prior to the 2016 elections!

Although it goes against popular belief for those living North of the Mason Dixon Line, there are Democrats living in Texas. One weekend in late October 2016, Sally, who was the senior GTCA camp counselor

---

[7] If you know where we can find any, please drop us a line!

for a group from Chicago, Illinois, was driving back to the ranch after a grocery run to Menard. She was an unhappy Sally as she would soon be out of range of Twitter, and therefore in her mind entering Hell. Before losing radio reception, Sally heard about a rally for her candidate in the metropolis of San Angelo and decided to attend. She drove as fast as she could up state highway, 83 then West on 87 to San Angelo, arriving at Rio Vista Park where the rally was in progress. As she walked toward the podium, several individuals greeted her with, "Mornin', ma'am," and "Howdy, miss." This irritated Sally to no end as she considered such greetings microaggressions. Furthermore, they were Texans, and she wanted nothing to do with them or their backwards *howdy* way of life!

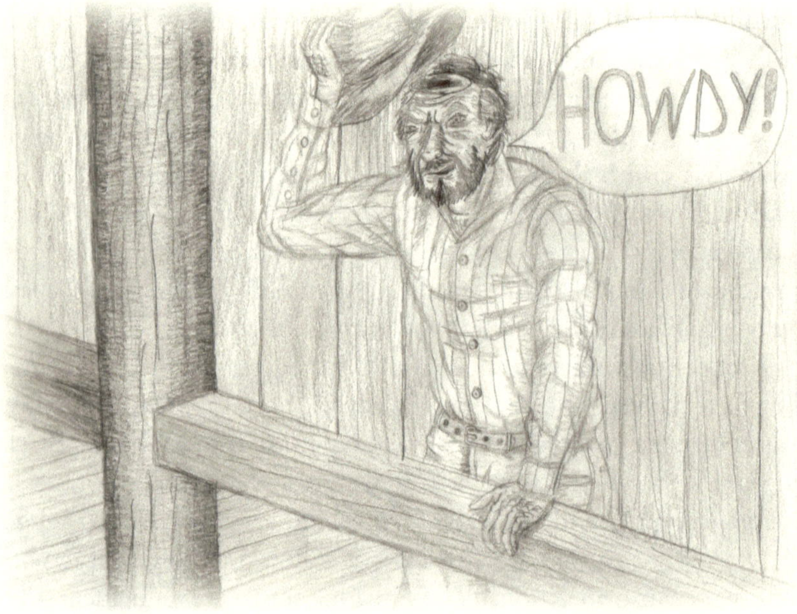

For forty minutes, the speakers told the crowd of twelve how their candidate would provide everything they required to survive: housing, food, cell phones, and connectivity! All twelve were cheering loudly when the podium was vacated and Sally decided to jump up and speak her mind! She looked down at the crowd and saw middle-aged women, Latinos, African Americans, and a Native American. As she began to tell the crowd about Northern progressive ideals, the clapping began to slow and become quieter. Apparently, Sally was unfamiliar with the term, *Blue Dog Democrat*. What happened next was witnessed by Buford Widerbutter, who provided the following statement to Menard County Sheriff, Buck Mueller, who was given jurisdiction because nobody else wanted to touch this case:

"I was sittin by what was left of last night's religious bonfire when I hear a young lady talkin' all suicidal-like! In front of a group of Texans, she begins talkin' bout guns killin' people, not people killin' people. Then she goes over the deep end and said if her candidate's elected, we'll rejoice in taking everyone's guns away and making ammunition illegal! It was with those statements that she committed suicide. Two little old ladies, one black and one white, pulled their matching pearl-handled P-33s with extended clips while the Native American and the Hispanic fellow whipped out their short guns (sawed-off 12 gauges). Then gay Jim whipped out his pistol and the shooting began. I figures there was at least fifty shots from just those folks, but I couldn't keep count of the shots from passersby's or those with long rifles and scopes on the rooftops who were huntin' squirrels."

Apparently, nobody at PSL Ranch had any idea that the GTCA camp counselor, Sally, was suicidal. An investigation was conducted in Chicago and police concluded that Sally's parents, friends, and siblings, all had similar suicidal thoughts, and that Sally should have never been allowed to become a GTCA counselor.

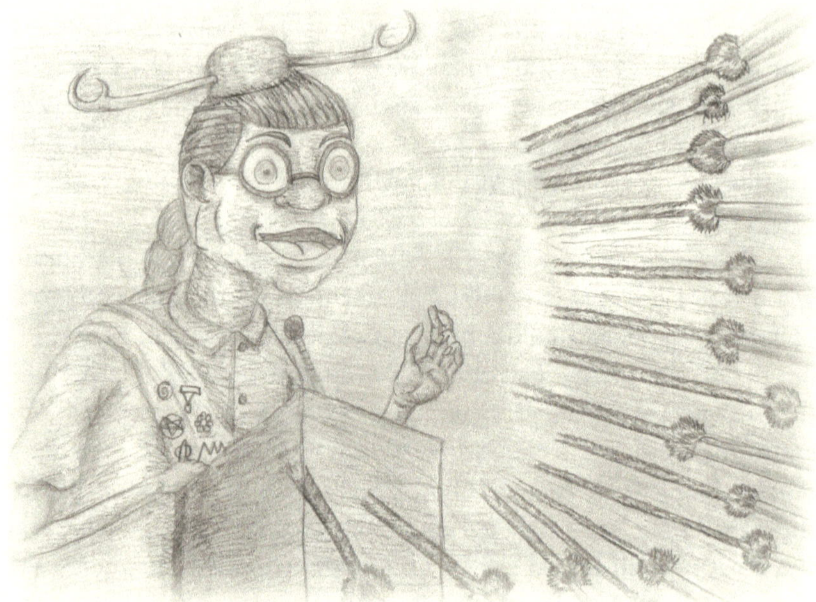

Menard County Sheriff, Buck Mueller, ruled the incident a *deplorable* suicide, and that PSL Ranch was not liable for the following reasons:

1. It was not PSL Ranch's responsibility to vet Sally for suicidal tendencies.
2. Sally committed suicide in a different county.
3. PSL Ranch was fined $25 for knowing about Sally's progressive tendencies and not shooting her locally; and for recruiting campers from Chicago in the first place!

As PSL Ranch attempts to appeal the fine (we're sending a $10 check to Judge Hangman's reelection campaign), we now provide a checklist of suicidal tendencies to all ranch hands and camp counselors so they will be alerted to warning signs:

Suicidal Thoughts	*Normal (Second Amendment) Thoughts*
The supreme court is wrong on the second amendment.	All citizens should be allowed to carry a weapon and protect themselves.
If the FBI is watching you, you shouldn't be able to just go buy a gun.	Repeal the Patriot Act!
Guns kill people, people don't kill people.	People kill people.
No one should be allowed to kill a deer.	Deer is good eatin'!
Hunting and trapping should be made illegal.	Hunting is in our nature, and a great outdoor activity.
Neil Young is a great singer.	Neil Young can't sing.
Country Western is not music!	There's music other than Country?

We at PSL Ranch believe this should help prevent future incidents like this one.

Conclusion: Know your audiences before you speak!

Hypothermia - A Winter Event

GTCA Camper Death Due to Improper Protection from Cold Temperatures

You've heard the saying, "If you don't like the weather, wait five minutes." This isn't one of those stories as it is almost always cold in Menard County in late January, and sometimes it even snows! In fact, unprotected water pipes can freeze from our winter weather as well as destroying peach crops and other fragile plants in our parcel of paradise.

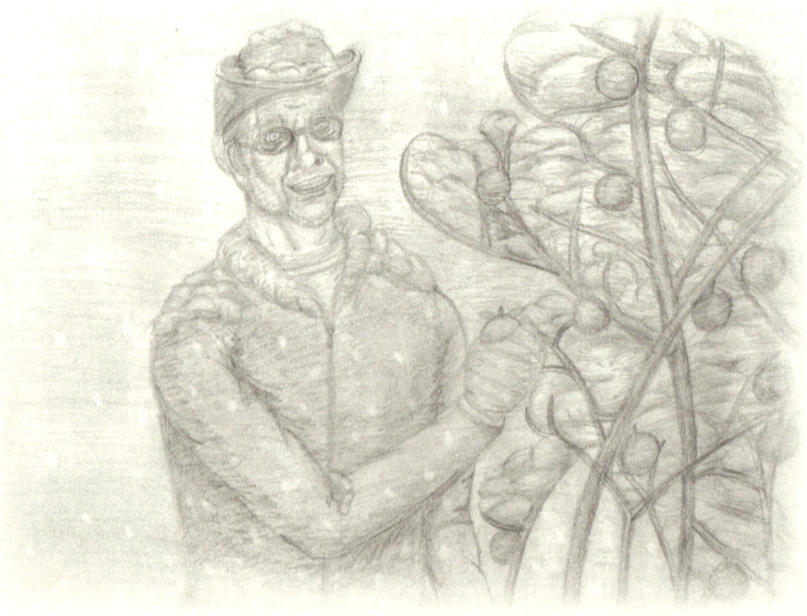

During a midwinter GTCA camping expedition to PSL Ranch, a group of young outdoor enthusiasts decided to spend a moonless-night stargazing with PSL Ranch's telescopes. It was a beautiful, cold, clear night with low humidity, and no light pollution—perfect for future astronomers to view the heavenly bodies. As the campers prepared to leave for the Eastern plains where there is a wide view of the sky, Cookie prepared her famous hot chocolate to keep them warm. What makes Cookie's hot chocolate famous? Most can't put their finger on it, but it may have something to do with the odor of schnapps wafting from the frothy brew.

As the campers filed out, Cassy called to one named Sally, "You nu see it cole out ear? Put on you jacket!" Sally simply smiled and continued out the door. What Cassy attempted to convey to Sally is that it was too cold to venture outside without proper protection against the environment, even with three of Cookie's hot chocolates in you! What happened that evening was documented in a testimonial provided to the Menard County sheriff's department by Funny Boy:

"I was helping Shari Running Wild with the stargazing that evening as our therapist thought it would be a good idea if we communicated in ways that didn't include racial slurs or lethal weapons. I was a little late getting to the camper's location because it was only 17 degrees Fahrenheit, and I had to layer up. When I finally got there, I heard Shari Running Wild detailing the constellations and other heavenly bodies to the eager campers."

Shari Running Wild, "There star. There star. There star. Funny Boy late."

Funny Boy continued, "Most everyone was feeling great after Cookie's hot chocolate, including some of the younger campers. One named Sally was feeling particularly good and was playing around with the others getting sweaty in her wool sweater, which she eventually took off and sat down to rest. Running Wild continued for another hour and a half, "There star. There star. There star," until we all got too cold because the wind had really picked up and we were out in the open. When we returned to the ranch house, Cookie was passed out, but her cocoa was still warm on the stove so we all had more until it was gone! The next afternoon, after we woke up and took medicine for our headaches, the camp counselors took roll and discovered Sally missing. Slim gave her scent to the ranch hound so he could track her down, but he refused to go outside (or even stand up) as the temperature outside was now only 10 degrees. After an hour of trying to get Cocoa to respond, we all went outside and found Sally frozen to the ground right where she fell asleep the night before! Dr. S said that when a body rapidly cools down, it could cause the person to go into hibernation. The only way to save them is to rapidly warm them, at least, that's what she thought they did on *Star Trek*? I suggested pouring boiling water over her for a rapid defrost the way Cookie does with the turkey every Thanksgiving. Slim wanted to put her on the spit over the campfire since she was too big to fit into the microwave or oven. Cookie suggested cutting off her little finger, "If she bleeds, she's still alive," she said; Cassy went to get her knife. It was then that Shari Running Wild sneezed. I jumped and let go of my end of the gurney that Sally was on. She fell hard on a large rock and shattered into a thousand pieces! What a skit this will make!"

Apparently, Cookie's hot chocolate had a magical effect on Sally, putting her in a deep sleep. The temps dropped rapidly to less than 10 degrees Fahrenheit, and the winds increased to twenty mph. By the time they reached poor little Sally, she was frozen from head to toe. When Funny Boy dropped her, she naturally cracked up!

Menard County Sheriff, Buck Mueller, ruled the incident a frosty demise and that PSL Ranch was not liable for the following reasons:

1. It was cold that night!
2. If Sally could have spoken Jamaican patois, she'd have known she was duly warned about the cold temperatures.
3. There was no hot chocolate left to analyze (Cookie drank the rest).

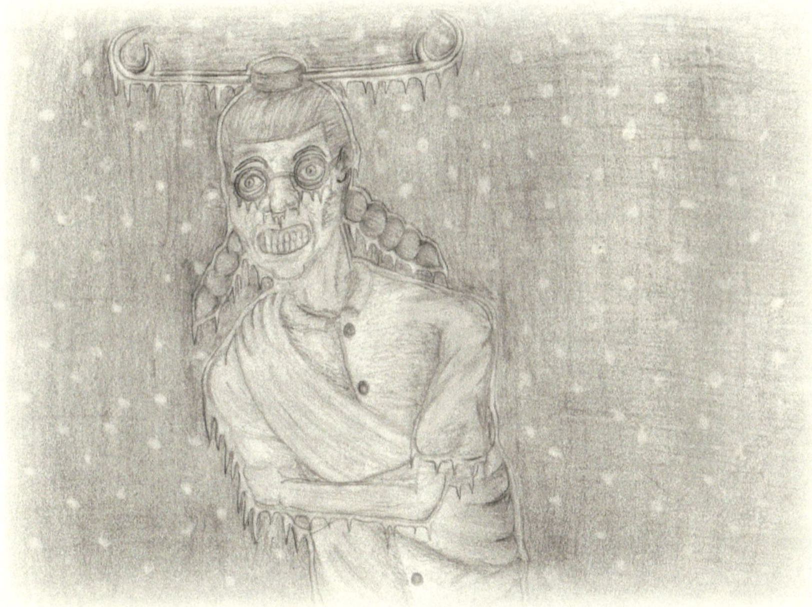

This incident gave us the shivers at PSL Ranch, and we decided to provide some facts about hypothermia to better educate campers and other visitors to this occasional winter wonderland:

- Hypothermia is defined as a body core temperature below 95.0 degrees Fahrenheit.
- Mild hypothermia causes shivering and mental confusion (ignore Slim, this is his natural state).
- During moderate hypothermia, the shivering stops and confusion increases.
- In severe hypothermia, victims may undress and there is an increased risk of the heart stopping.
- Hypothermia can also occur from any condition that decreases heat production or increases heat loss such as alcohol consumption.
- During Napoleon Bonaparte's retreat from Russia in the winter of 1812, many troops died from hypothermia.

- An average of 1,301 people die from hypothermia annually in the United States.
- It can get very cold in Central Texas.

We hope these facts can prevent future ice cubing of campers by increasing the knowledge of our visitors.

Conclusion: If you drink Cookie's hot chocolate, stay by the campfire!

Blue Wildebeest and Nilgai Blue Bull: They're Not Cattle

Goring of a GTCA Camper

Although they are rarely found on PSL Ranch, large-horned exotic animals do visit our location from time to time, and they are a sight to behold! The wildebeest and Nigali blue bull were introduced to Texas hunting ranches in the 1930s, and many have escaped to roam the countryside. Today, the majority are confined to the Edwards Plateau region, also known as the Texas Hill country where we are located, but an estimated seventy-four thousand animals are free-range, meaning they are free to travel between ranches.

These are *wild* animals, not tame or friendly in anyway. They may be aggressive and are usually on their guard as most are considered intrusive to natural wildlife and can be hunted year-round. Unfortunately, one GTCA camper named Sally discovered this the hard way.

On a crisp fall morning, the silence at PSL Ranch was broken by several faraway gun shots. There are many hunting ranches located in Menard and surrounding counties, so this is a common sound at our location aside from Cassy yelling at Slim to get to work. Several of the GTCA campers wanted to take a quick hike to the Eastern edge of the property to see if the raccoons who wrecked their campsite the evening before were still in the vicinity. One of the campers, Sally, took a stick to whack them if she could get close enough as they ate all of her cupcakes. As the campers strolled over the prairie, they passed some cattle lazily strolling and eating grass. The herd that

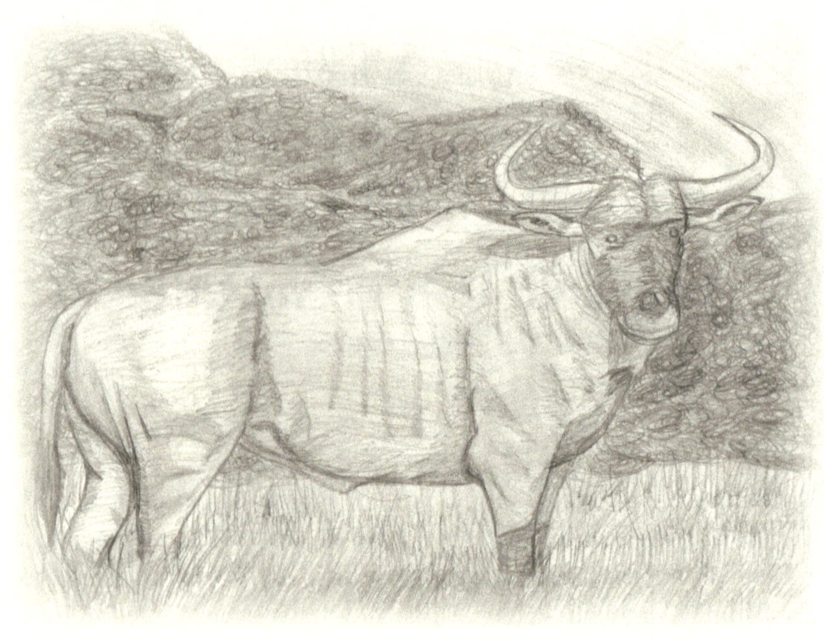

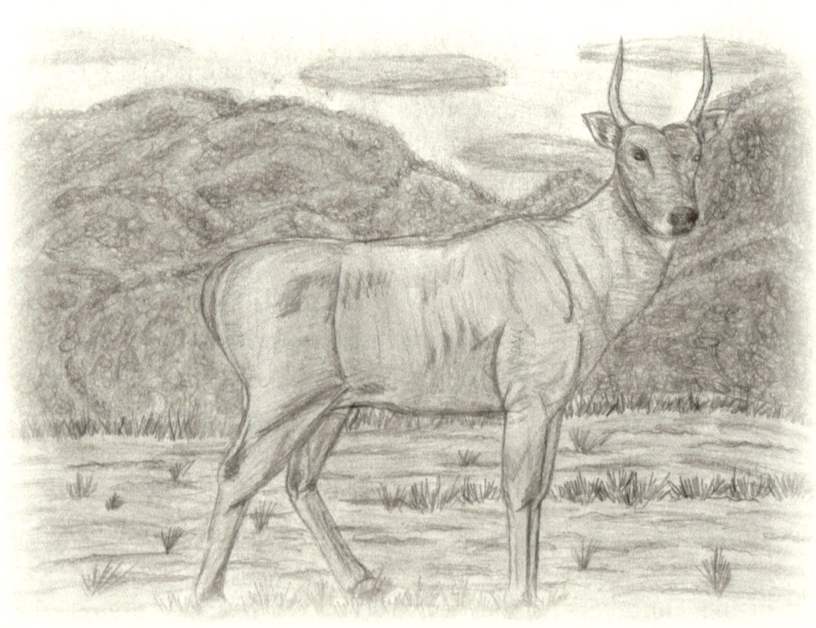

visits PSL Ranch is usually docile and ignores campers as they pass closely by. Suddenly, a large cow-like animal broke the herd up and stopped in its tracks directly in front of the campers. Sally, being a pesky child, decided if she couldn't whack a raccoon she would whack the cow thingy in her path. What happened next was witnessed by Dr. S who happened to be investigating strange markings in nearby stones that she found interesting. The following testimonial was provided to the Menard County sheriff's department:

"I was watching TV the night before and learned that aliens may have built the pyramids in Egypt. Many of the markings on the walls were like those on some limestone outcroppings at PSL Ranch, and I wanted to be the first to definitively prove cowboys were put on earth by extraterrestrials. I believed this would launch my career and prove to my peers at the University of Chicago that I'm not a crackpot Archeologist! Anyway, while I was examining the rocks, I looked up and saw this little camper whacking a huge wildebeest in the face with a short stick! My first thought was, *what an idiot*! I then saw the animal jump forward and launch her into the air. As it began to run away from the camper, Sally [I think was her name] landed right on the large horns. It began to run back the way it came and was never seen again—neither was Sally."

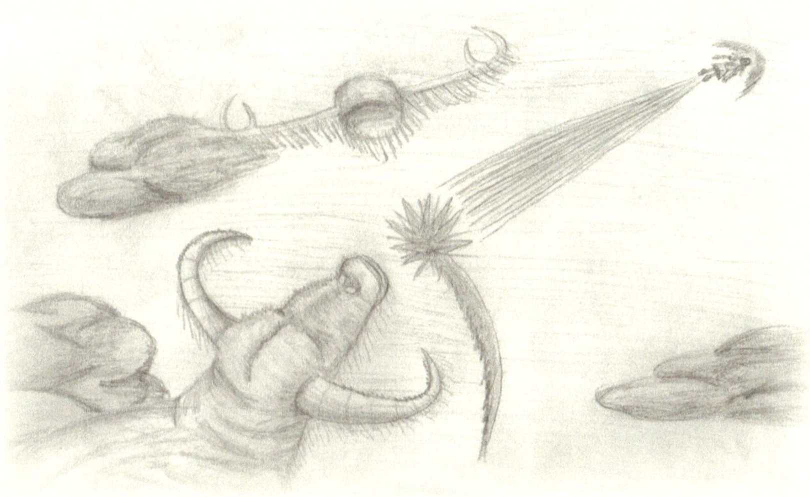

Apparently, the animal was running from hunters and was terribly agitated when it arrived at PSL Ranch. Sally's attempt to whack it further irritated the poor animal who, feeling threatened, gored and ran away with poor Sally on its horns. Slim took some of Sally's clothes for the scent and gave the ranch hound a sniff so he could track her and the wildebeest. After several hours of inactivity, Cocoa got up and walked over to Cookie's stove. It appears Cookie used Sally's cloths as a dish cloth the night before to clean her pots.

Menard County Sheriff Buck Mueller pointed out that this incident was a sticky issue, but that PSL Ranch was not liable for the following reasons:

1. Although you can hunt wildebeest year-round in Menard County, whacking season was still two months off.
2. Again, you must have a body before there is a crime.
3. Cookie's cooking will kill the scent of anything, so there was nothing more to be done.

A further investigation was conducted to see if the chili made the night before had any traces of Sally in it, but after two bowls, Sheriff Mueller concluded the meat used wasn't Sally; although, what was used was never determined.[8]

Conclusion: Don't whack a wildebeest unless you're absolutely sure you can get away with it!

---

[8] No PSL ranch hand has eaten Cookie's chili since this incident.

INCIDENT #37

Cattle: They Are Dumb Animals!
Stampede Death of a GTCA Camper

Bovine, or cattle as they are commonly known, are large animals that spend their lives eating grass, hay, and grains until they reach an age and size where ranchers take them to market. They are then transported to packing plants where they are chopped up, ground up, and processed into tasty morsels of protein for humans to consume.

During the early years of the Western migration into Central Texas, to include Menard County and other surrounding counties, famous ranchers such as John Chisum and Richard Tankersley had enormous herds of cattle that roamed the open range. These ranchers didn't necessarily own all of the land, but rather had rights to it for their cattle to graze on. They would round them up on a yearly basis, separate them by brands, and conduct a common trail ride to the closest stockyards—sometimes as far as San Bernardino, California in Tankersley's case! It was a wild time to live in Menard County as the cattle and sheep wars took place among those vying for land and pasture. Cattle rustling was big business with the likes of Jessie James and Tom (Black Jack) Ketchum (a local train robber), who stole from both Chisum and Tankersley.

If you drive around Menard County's countryside today, you'll see cattle gates crossing the ranch roads to separate herds. The open range still exists to a certain extent as cattle will block the road on occasion while crossing from one ranch to the next. PSL Ranch is part of a larger open range for a herd of Black Angus cattle that roam for miles around, but still seem to deposit their poop (cow pies) directly in front of our ranch house's back porch steps. Furthermore, they think they own the place and will not move out of the way of your Jeep or truck, let alone some hikers!

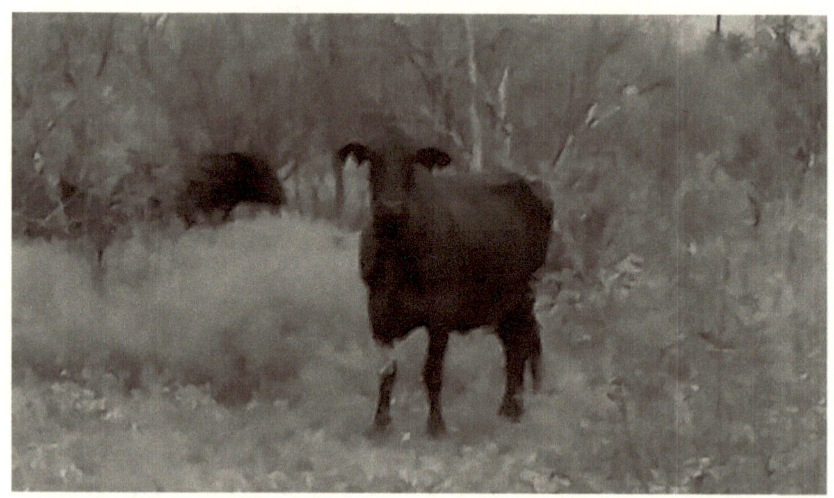

A couple of PSL Ranch's herd lurking behind the ranch house

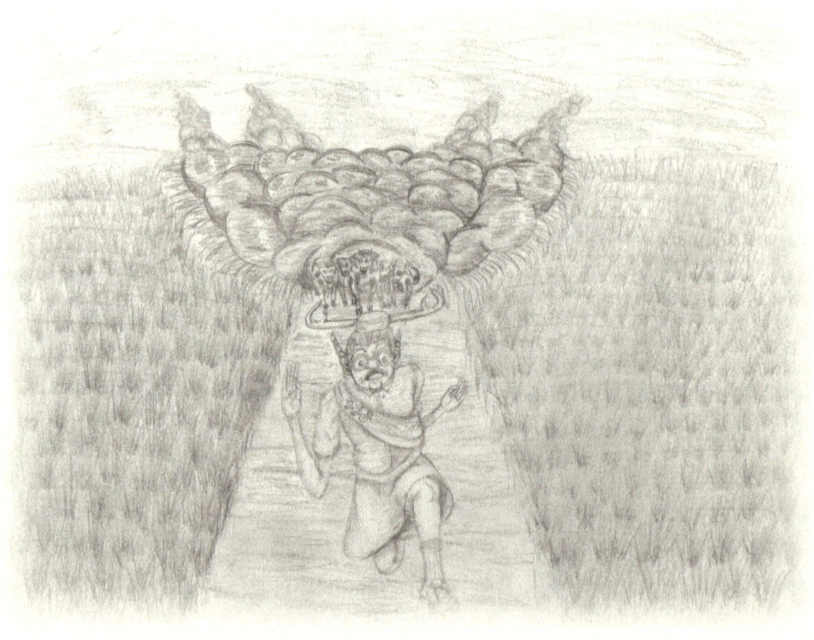

One late spring day, a group of GTCA hikers were traveling to the Western boundary of PSL ranch to observe a family of gray foxes. Unfortunately, the only approved trail that crossed the wash was occupied by twenty to twenty-five cattle who were stopping for a drink of wash water. They had just finished eating all of the corn at the deer feeder and were heading back to poop on the ranch house steps. Usually, hikers only have to wait for a few minutes before the cattle move on, but on this day the cattle were in no hurry as they had several young calves accompanying them and their mothers were being protective. This irritated one camper named Sally, who being ignorant in the way of bovines, took a short stick and began running at the cattle yelling for them to move. What followed was witnessed by Slim who happened to be across the wash cutting down some small trees:

"I was cuttin' down sum short pole trees to make stilts for our little campers so they don't have to feel so short. Every now and then we gits one of them dwarves or midgets[9] who are always lagging behind or jumpin' up to see what's goin' on. So I thinks, if I put them on stilts they's be like everyone else! Of course, them little dwarf fellas tend to waddle, so I cut one of their stilts a little shorter to compensate.[10] Anyway, as I was cuttin' away, I saw one of them campers with the funny hats wackin' one of the old cows with a stick. That old cow didn't move much until the camper, Sally was her name, wacked the old girl's calf in the head with a stick and it began to baller! Right then, the old girl ran at Sally at full steam and the rest of the herd followed behind until they reached the ranch house. All the campers leaped out of the way into the cactus and mesquite, except one. Poor, little, Sally. She could've used my stilts today!"

[9.] PSL ranch hands no longer refer to midgets or dwarfs as midgets and dwarfs, as we have been informed by our legal staff that those terms can be offensive, even if they are accurate. Therefore, we only use terms such as wee little people. Short shits, shrimps, half-pints, and similar politically correct descriptors as defined by the Wee People of America organization.

[10.] Slim's experiment went horribly wrong. Stilts are no longer used on PSL Ranch.

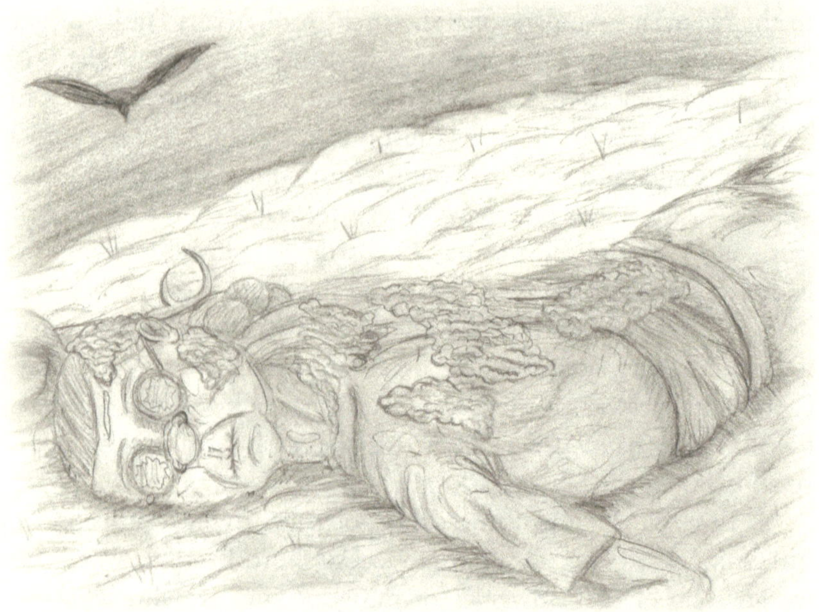

Menard County Sheriff, Buck Mueller, ruled the stampede self-inflicted, and PSL Ranch not liable for the following reasons:

1. Sally instigated the stampede by hitting the poor little calf in the head.
2. Everyone else got out of the way, therefore, Sally could have.
3. Menard County Statute A-207 clearly states that hitting a calf in the head is tantamount to rustling, and the offender should be hanged, found guilty, and prosecuted in that order.
4. Because the resulting stampede killed Sally, no further action was necessary by county officials.

This momentous bad luck could have been avoided if Sally had just watched the movie *Red River* starring John Wayne. Therefore, to prevent future issues involving trampled children and cow poop, PSL ranch administrators have published a few rules and facts for visitors that should make their stay safer and more enjoyable:

1. Don't hit calves (or cows) in the head with a stick, that's just plain mean.
2. Don't even approach the cattle or harass them in anyway, unless they are pooping on the porch steps, in which case you tell Cassy—she'll handle them!
3. Cows get mean if their calves are threatened.
4. Cows are dumb animals that weigh over one thousand pounds—they will crush you by accident!
5. Cows do not talk like the California milk commercials pretend they do, and therefore cannot be reasoned with; Californians are dumb animals too.
6. Don't step in the cow pies and walk in the ranch house.
7. Cattle have been known to deliberately attack people. The CDC estimates approximately twenty-two people were killed by cows in a three-year period, and of those cow attacks, 75 percent were known to be non-provoked attacks.[11]

PSL Ranch authorities hope these simple, easy to remember, and understandable facts will help visitors to our property have a safe time while strolling around.

Conclusion: Don't whack the calves!

[11.] http://www.cdc.gov/mmwr/preview/mmwrhtml/mm5829a2.html

Singing Southern Man on Karaoke Night at Uncle Weirdo's Tavern

Another Appalling Suicide by a GTCA Camp Coordinator

After a hard day of punching cattle, processing deer, and watching the Veterans Day parade in Menard, Texas, many of the cowboys, cowgirls, and long-time residents like to relax at Uncle Weirdo's Tavern for some cold beer and karaoke. Charlie Daniels, Neil Diamond, Brittney Spears, and the Village People are crowd favorites, especially when sung by one of PSL's ranch hands. These fun-loving and hardworking folks come from all backgrounds and lifestyles, but one thing they all have in common is a love for their town and their way of life.

Following one cantankerous week of GTCA campers that included bee stings, a localized fire, lost campers (we found most), and lots of crying children wanting to go home, one GTCA camp coordinator named Sally wanted to get away for a while and have a cold beer. Sally was a GTCA volunteer from Redman Washington who worked as a programmer for Macrosoft, a massive software company with the logo, *Our software doesn't always work, but it's expensive!* She volunteered as a camp coordinator as a means to give back to the community and to show her employer that she is compassionate and worthy of a promotion. Many large corporations encourage their employees to do community projects, and Sally was filling a square in her resume for advancement. Unfortunately, not everyone is cut out for community service, and Sally was one that should have worked a soup kitchen rather than try to herd children. She was frazzled and at her wit's end when she arrived at Uncle Weirdo's that evening and the karaoke stage became available. What happened next was witnessed by Cassy who had just finished her rendition of *Country Roads*:

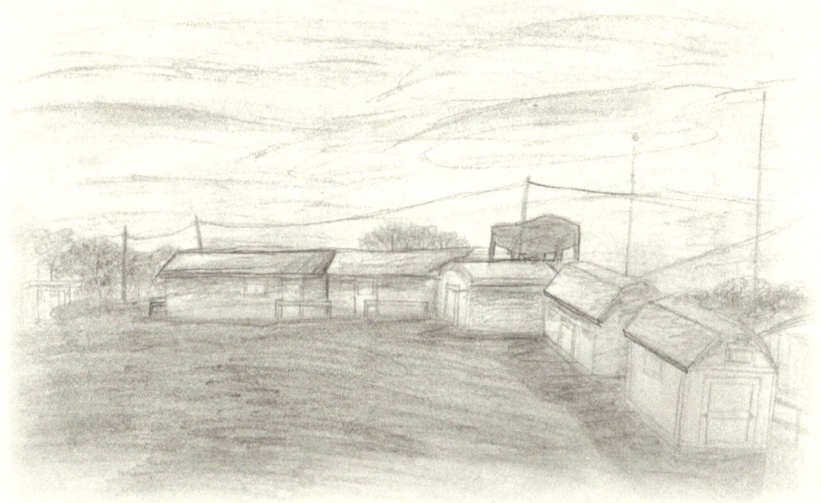

"Sally jump pon di stage an she staht to sing. She sing awrite, but are chaiese of song was awful: Neil Young's *Soudern Man*! At fers di bar go quiet, but when she sing, 'Soudern change gonna come at lass," di young gal lite up like a light bulb an she drop ded!"

Apparently, Sally got the cold beer she wanted as several beers were tossed from the crowd landing on her microphone, which sent several thousand volts through her. This caused the circuit breakers to click off, and the whole place went dark. By the time the lights came back on, Sally was lying on the stage stiff as a board. An investigation was conducted to find out who threw the beer, but it was never determined. It might have been one of the cowboys sitting in the back, but cowboys in this area would never waste a good beer. It may have been one of the ladies from the Holy Cross Church assembly who were sitting in the front row, but their average age is ninety-three, and they were mostly drinking scotch on the rocks. The Menard County sheriff's department tried looking at the video recordings from security cameras around Uncle Weirdo's Tavern, but they were running on Macrosoft software and not working.

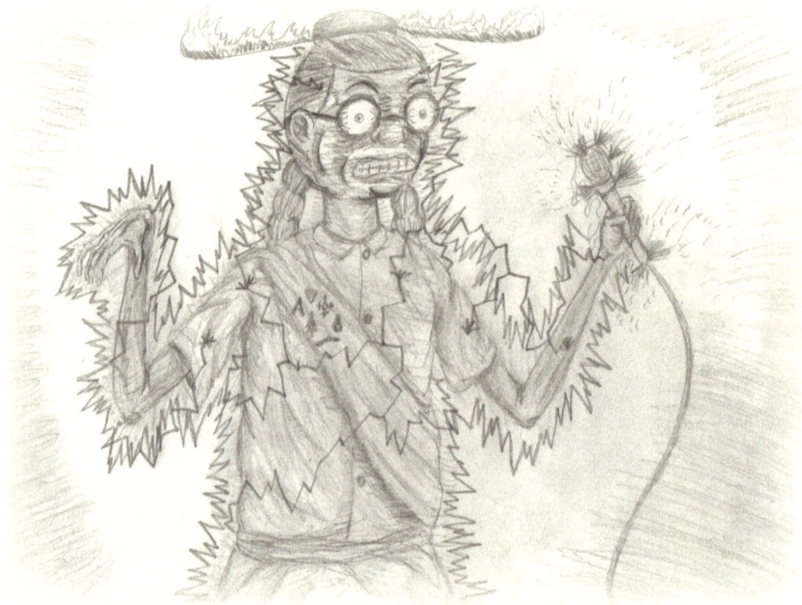

Menard County Sheriff, Buck Mueller, ruled the incident another GTCA suicide, and Uncle Weirdo's Tavern not liable for the following reasons:

1. Sally obviously wanted to end it all with a song like that.
2. If it was one of the old church ladies, it was an act of God.
3. Shame about the wasted beers!

Cassy felt bad about the incident and felt somewhat responsible for not briefing Sally and the other camp coordinators of cultural differences they might find in our Central Texas community. Slim always wondered what happened to the three beers Cassy had in front of her prior to the incident. Therefore, PSL Ranch now provides a list of acceptable and safe songs that can be sung at Uncle Weirdo's on karaoke night:

- *Swamp Witch*
- *Long-Haired Country Boy*
- *Take Back the USA*
- *Copperhead Road*
- *Country Boys Can Survive*
- *Rawhide*
- *Riders in the Sky*

PSL Ranch would like to look at this incident as a learning opportunity. From now on, at least two ranch hands must accompany Cassy whenever she attends karaoke night at Uncle Weirdo's Tavern.

Conclusion: Know what the lyrics are before you sing a song!

Incident #39

Skeeters by the Millions!

Death of a GTCA Camper Due to Blood Loss

Imagine being alone on a remote part of PSL Ranch near dusk. The sun nearly out of sight as the sound of hundreds of thousands of toads and frogs begin to rise in volume until your screams for help are drowned out. You become silent as you begin to realize the creature that you were warned about begins to stalk you; *Bzzzz* is all you can hear!

At this point, if you're smart, you'll add a little more DEET to your exposed skin or roll down your long sleeves to prevent multiple bites! Yes, you've guessed it, the creature after your blood is no other than the dreaded mosquito (skeeters for the locals). The loud sounds from the toads and frogs should alert most that there is a healthy mosquito population on PSL Ranch, as skeeters are the amphibian's favorite early-morning and late-afternoon snack.

As part of PSL Ranch's ten-hour safety briefing, Slim and Cassy warn guests and campers that these pesky little creatures love to bite humans since most of the time they can only feed from thick cow and deer hides. It seems they particularly like guests on our ranch! For some odd reason, those that visit are bitten more often; although, this may be to the local's unconscious ability to take preventive actions or stay in the cabin during peak skeeter hours. Skeeters smell blood through the skin organ, and those with thin skin are sure to be skewered multiple times if not protected. In fact, thin clothing alone will not protect one from the little monsters, so applying mosquito repellent to thin clothing is also recommended!

One hot spring day a group of GTCA campers were preparing for a night of astronomy, a favorite activity at PSL Ranch which provides some of the clearest skies in North America. About a week prior, heavy rains to the area left about a foot of water at the bottom of the wash, which of course was renamed Lake Rohret.

Previously, Slim and Cassy noticed a marked increase in skeeters and provided every camper with DEET; advising them to wear long-sleeved shirts and full-length pants to prevent multiple bites. One GTCA camper, named Sally, was a naturalist and decided not to put the evil chemical on her skin. Furthermore, due to the high temperature and her desire to show-off her legs to a boy that caught her fancy, Sally decided to wear a tank top and short-shorts.

As the group prepared to depart by smearing repellant over every inch of their bodies, Sally took off early to the viewing location in order to admire the clear skies as the sun descended over the far horizon. What happened next was witnessed by Cassy who happened to be a couple of hundred yards away collecting milkweed for some reason:

"Mi was listening to di naise di frog an' toad a mek as dem was eatin' di masquito, when mi tink mi ear a chile scream. So mi a look aad inna di direction a di naise, when mi si a gal pickney a run roun', flapping are arms all 'bout like she crazy. All of a sudden, she fly up inna di air and drop… *babs*! Mi tink to miself… *Laad Ga… a wha' dat*? Mi was fearful dat di spirits dat did lif' di chile up would catch mi to, so mi tek time an walk ova deh. Mi catch mi fright when mi si masquito tree feet tick, but no pickney! Mi no believe what mi a si! Ida Cookie brew nuh good, are obeah deh! Ida way, mi nah stay deer. Mi tek ahf an' run back to di kyabin as fas' as mi could goh."

English Translation: I heard the frogs and toads begin to make noise as they began to feed on the skeeters. Then I heard a scream and saw a camper running in circles waving her arms. I thought I saw her lifted off of the ground and thought, *what magic is this*! I walked over to the location of the screams and saw a pile of skeeters but no camper. I thought Cookie's home brew was causing my hallucinations and returned to the ranch house for help.

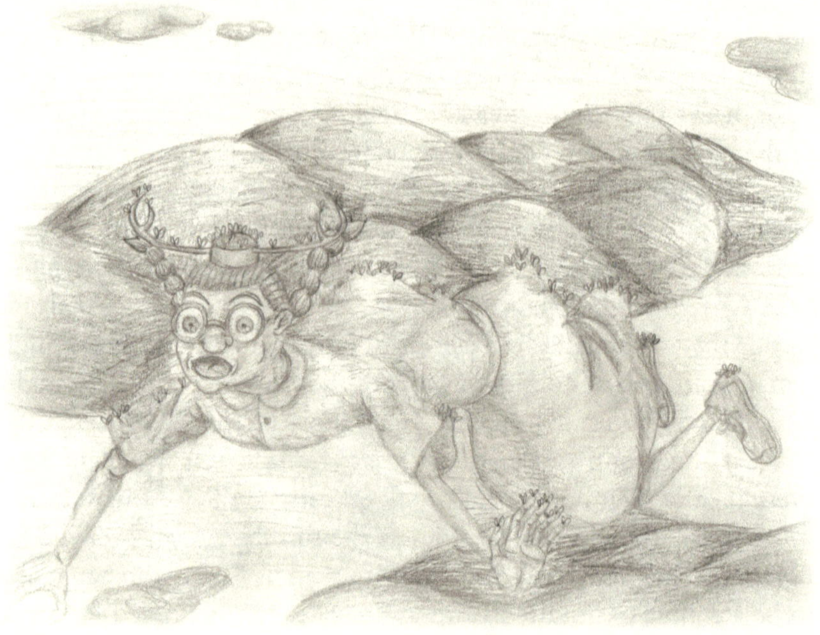

Once back at the ranch house, Cassy conveyed her story to Slim, who then told Cookie, who then told Funny Boy, who then told Dr. S, who then asked Shari Running Wild to investigate. After lathering up with DEET, Shari Running Wild left for the location to find a lifeless body drained of blood lying by a telescope. The body was identified as Sally by Dr. S from the short-shorts and a tank top.

Apparently, Sally had walked into a major swarm of Culex mosquitos that were very hungry, and she panicked!

Menard County Sheriff, Buck Mueller, ruled the incident a natural event, and PSL Ranch was not liable for the following reasons:

1. Sally was warned about the danger of Skeeters and offered protection.
2. Sally chose not to protect herself.
3. It was a natural way to go!

PSL Ranch views this incident as one shrouded in stupidity! Still, administrators decided to provide some facts about the Central Texas mosquito population to those visiting our piece of utopia to help prevent future incidents like this one:

- The month of April is the beginning of our skeeter season.
- Texas mosquitos do not carry the Zika virus (yet).
- There are 3,500 species of skeeters, but Texas has only about 85 different kinds.
- The Culex mosquito carries the West Nile Virus, which is known to be in Texas.
- According to the World Health Organization, mosquitos are the deadliest animal in the world killing an average of 1 million worldwide annually.
- There have been cases of individuals dying from shock due to hundreds of mosquito bites in a short period.
- Using insect repellent when going outside and wearing long sleeves at dawn and dusk when skeeters are most active is the best prevention against being bitten.

Conclusion: Don't be a naturalist on PSL Ranch!

Don't Worry - There Are No Bears or Wolves on PSL Ranch Yet!

The Center for Biological Diversity reported[12] that Texas is one of the top-four states where the USDA's Wildlife Service has killed the largest number of black bears, mountain lions, wolves, and bobcats in 2015 to protect humans, livestock, and property. This has been a turnaround in the last twenty or so years as all species of bears and wolves that used to roam the Texas hills and plains were eliminated by hunters in the 1920s and 1970s respectively.

Concerning Bears: A long time ago, two species of bears were numerous in Texas: black bears and brown (grizzly) bears. Grizzly bears were heavily hunted from the mid-nineteenth century through nineteen-twenty, at which time they were eliminated from the Texas countryside. The Eastern Black Bear was hunted out by nineteen-twenty as well. Bears were coveted by Native Americans and early white settlers as a food source and for their furs, which brought a good price in European markets. Later, as ranchers and farmers began to encroach on their habitat, they became a danger to livestock and settlers, and were eliminated. Hunting bears were some men's passion, such as Texas Liberty County Judge Lewis Hightower, who reportedly killed two hundred bears in the late eighteen-hundreds earning him the nickname, the Bear Hunting Judge. Hightower was quoted as saying, "I practice law for recreation and hunt bear for a livin'."[13]

---

[12] http://texashillcountry.com/texas-killed-bears-mountain-lions-wolves/.
[13] https://tshaonline.org/handbook/online/articles/fhi63.

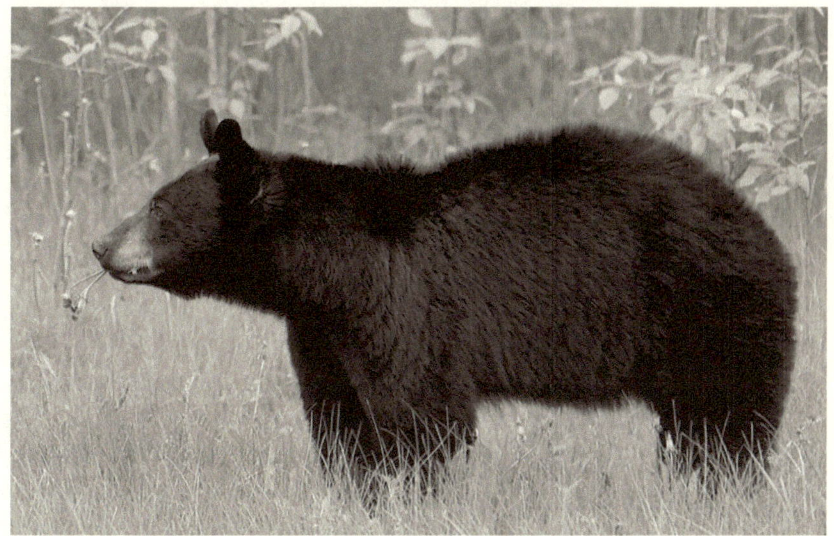

Black Bear[14]

In 1983, black bears began creeping back into Texas, and the state legislature outlawed hunting them that same year. Since then, black bears are routinely spotted crossing the Red River and Sabine River returning to their natural habitat. In 2009, on a twelve-thousand-acre Menard County ranch, Chief Broken Eagle, a descendant of the Tonkawa Indians of Central Texas, spotted a black bear. This sighting was confirmed by the Texas parks and wildlife agency, proving black bears are now in our county! At the time this conservation and safety guide was published, PSL Ranch hands had not spotted any bears on our property. Texas lists the black bear as threatened, and the penalty for shooting one is a class *C* misdemeanor with a fine of $500 plus a civil restitution of $11,907.50.[15] Still, landowners have the right to protect livestock and human life.

Concerning Wolves: At one time, there were two species of wolves in Texas: the Southeastern red wolf (Canis rufus), and the once more widespread gray wolf (Canis lupus). Gray wolves were hunted to extinction in Texas by 1970, and the red wolves became

---

[14.] Courtesy of pixabay.com/en/bear-animal-nature-wild-fur-1102599.

[15.] We have no idea why this sum was chosen!

so scarce that they began breeding with coyotes. By 1980, there were only seventeen red wolves remaining without coyote DNA. Texas now is participating in a program where red wolves are being reintroduced to the Texas wilderness. Red wolves are smaller than their gray cousins and have a reddish tint in their lower bodies and head. They can also be black-and-tan in color, making them difficult to discern from coyotes. PSL Ranch hand, Slim, has spotted a large coyote-looking animal with red legs and head, but he stated it could have been an unusually large gray fox, therefore, it cannot be determined that PSL Ranch has any wolves roaming around at this time. Still, it would be a good idea to remain vigilant when roaming around areas of PSL Ranch with lots of jack rabbits, which are one of the wolves' favorite food sources.

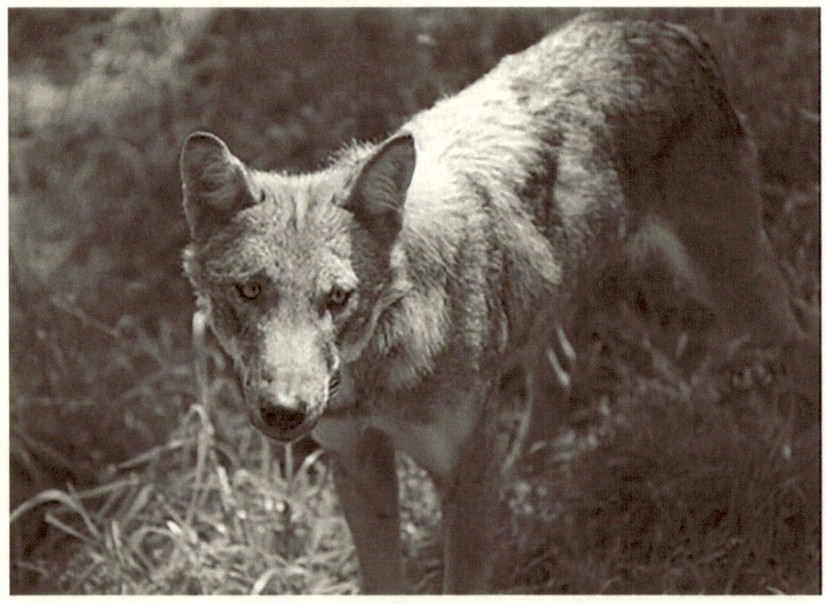

Red Wolf[16]

---

16. Courtesy of https://pixabay.com/en/wolf-zoo-cute-predator-deer-park-1621456/.

What do you do if you see a black bear or red wolf? Both can be aggressive animals, particularly if you come between them and their young or their food.

If you happen to run into Chief Broken Eagle's black bear, the conventional wisdom is to hold your ground and don't run. The following tips may save your life:

- Stop, stay calm and quiet, and make no sudden moves.
- Do not stare directly into the bear's eyes, as this is a sign of aggression.
- Stand your ground and do not turn your back on the bear.
- Back away slowly, speaking in a calming, monotone voice to show the bear you are being submissive and want to get out of its territory.
- If the bear comes at you, spray it in the face with bear mace.
- Keep a cool head—try to stay calm, do not yell or scream.
- If all else fails, shoot it!

Preventing a wolf attack is a bit different; the following tips may save your life!

- Don't run!
- Don't stare the animal down.
- Don't turn your back on the wolf or wolves.
- Make yourself appear scary: shout, throw stones, and raise your arms over your head.
- If you've entered an enclosure, back away slowly, moving toward the exit with your back against the fence or rock wall.
- Don't look scared or fall, this will encourage an attack.
- If all else fails, shoot!

Now don't you feel better? Of course, other animals aren't so easily spooked. The mountain lion, which does visit PSL Ranch from time to time, is a formidable hunter and PSL ranch hands provide the following tips for survival if you were to stumble on this lovable cat:

- Avoid any dead animal that could be a cougar kill—they don't like to share!
- Travel in a group.
- Keep small children and anyone named Sally within reach—mountain lions will watch and wait for an opportunity to grab a child.
- Carry a walking stick; it could be used in your defense.
- If you see one, yell and scream—intimidate it as a fierce predator!
- If all else fails, shoot it!

As with the other large predators that could eat you, it's best you travel in groups and have some form of defense with you such as a gun and a walking stick. No one has actually been attacked on PSL Ranch to date, but we strongly advise vigilance and avoid hiking with Sally!

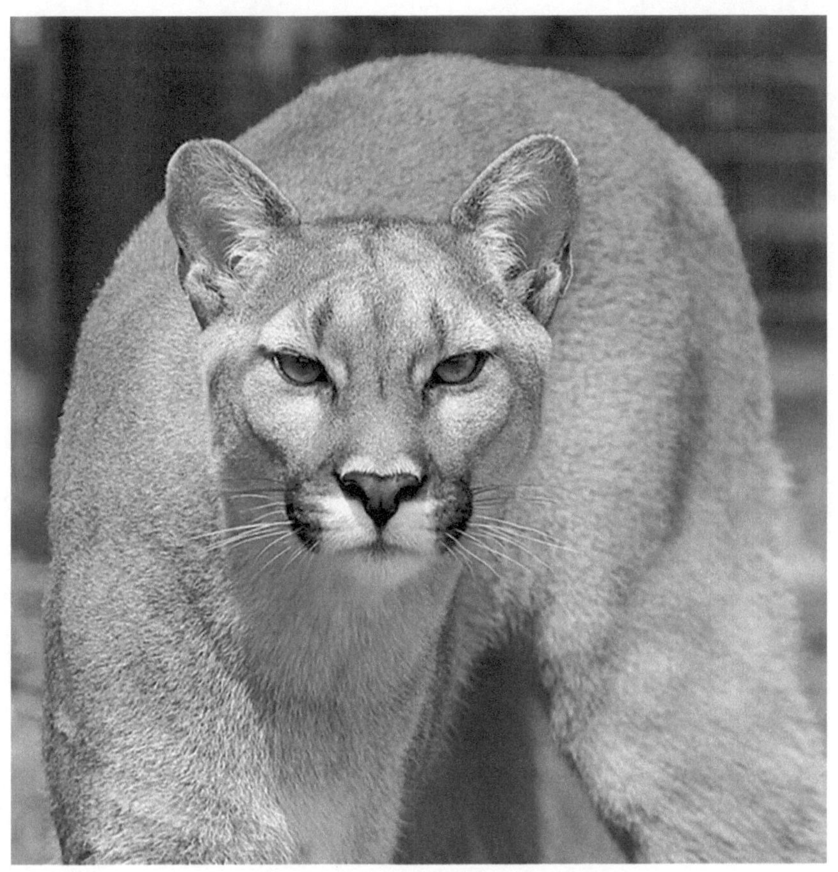

Mountain Lion (Cougar)[17]

[17.] Courtesy of https://pixabay.com/en/cougar-mountain-lion-pumqa-concolor-275945/.

Epilogue

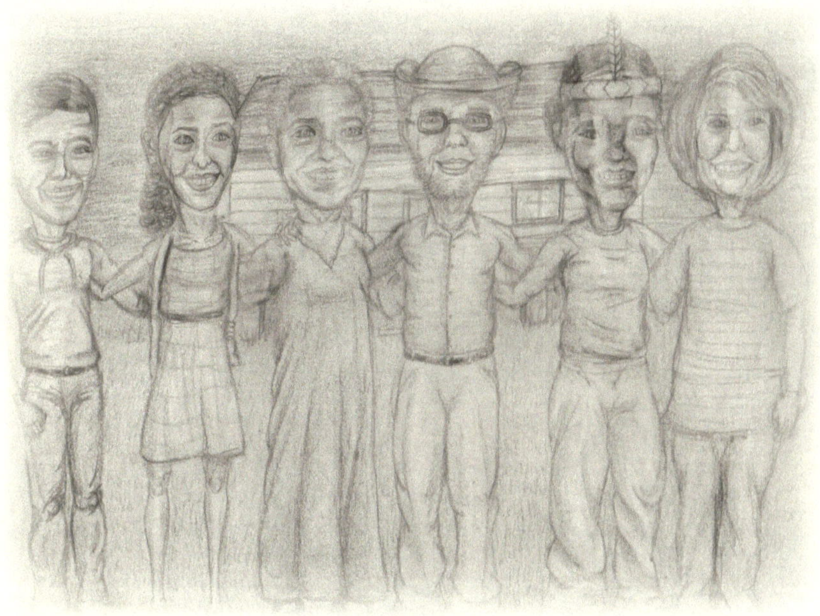

Slim and Cassy still maintain PSL Ranch, providing a wonderful camping and hiking experience for those who want to enjoy the beauty of the Central Texas countryside.

Shari Running Wild can be spotted roaming around the ranch creating wonderful 2.4 percent Native American trinkets for our visitors to purchase at an extremely high price. She is often seen practicing her archery using a picture of Funny Boy.

Funny Boy still visits PSL Ranch on occasion, mostly to see what is going to happen to Sally so he can create more hilarious skits for his audiences. His visits coincide with Shari Running Wild's time away from the ranch.

Dr. S spends much of her time in Egypt attempting to prove that civilization began there as an alien experiment from some distant planet. She does return to PSL Ranch on occasion to study Shari Running Wild in the wild, and to sample Cookie's home brew.

Cookie still enjoys scaring children around the campfire and operates one of the largest illegal moonshine stills in the Southwest. Her world-famous cuisine is enjoyed by travelers from all over the world especially the French, who are accustomed to eating snails, pressed raw duck, and other animal parts no decent, bathing American would eat.

Cocoa, the ranch hound, has retired to the city. Now over seventeen years old, mostly deaf and blind. His smell and ability to walk has greatly decreased. Cocoa still gets his fill of steak and table scraps, and seems to be happy![18]

[18.] At the time of publication, Cocoa has departed the living and now resides in a beautiful oak box on a mantel in the PLS Ranch cabin. Doggie-B-Gone was not used in his internment.

Book a Camping Site at PSL Ranch

Due to several recent incidents involving GTCA campers on PSL Ranch, there are now many openings for those daring outdoorsmen and women wishing to explore the wilds of Central Texas. Reserving a campsite is simple, just follow the directions below.

Provide the date(s) you wish to camp. Providing alternate dates in case your primary date is unavailable.

Provide proof of health insurance. This is a formality only as you will be so far from any hospital; it's doubtful you would survive long enough to reach a hospital in the event of a serious accident.

Provide proof of funeral insurance notarized by three notary officers. If you are unable to complete this requirement prior to arriving at PSL Ranch, local funeral homes can provide your insurance needs and it won't break your budget.

Provide a $1,000,000.00 bond in case of accident ($2,000,000.00 if your name is Sally) notarized by three notary officers. If your state prohibits you from acquiring a bond for personnel injury, don't fret, PSL Ranch can provide the bond for a nominal fee.

Send a deposit of $5000 in Bitcoin or foreign currency (all deposits are non-refundable). The current price of Bitcoins is $7,554.73 per coin! That means your deposit is only about three-fifths of a coin! Where can you buy Bitcoins, create a Bitcoin Wallet, and transfer Bitcoins to our off-shore account? That's what Google is for!

Sign our two-hundred-fifty-page disclaimer written in the Navajo language. No, Shari Running Wild doesn't speak Navaho, or any other Native American Language for that matter. We believe this disclaimer adds an ambiance to the entire process that fits our *Old West* experience. Besides, the legalese in English is just as unintelligible.

PSL Recipes

PSL Ranch has been inundated with requests for our world-famous recipes, and we are obliging with a full-sized cookbook in the near future, but to give you a taste of what's to come, here are a few of our best camper meals and snacks!

Cookie's Potato Soup

This hearty soup will fill your guest's gullet to the brim! Cookie calls this her 5-5-5 tater recipe, and it will serve up to fifty campers squealing with hunger!

Ingredients:

> 5 pounds of milk thistle (plant heads
> with 5 inches of the lower stalk). *Do
> not* use milkweed as a substitute!
> 5 pounds of salted butter (no sub-
> stitution allowed)
> two-gallon cans of generic store-bought
> potato soup (any brand will do,
> Cookie uses the cheapest)
> 5 pints of moonshine
> 5 ounces of black pepper

Step 1: The first step is to send your equivalent of Funny Boy out into the thistle patch to pick the milk thistle. Once he/she/it returns, throw the milk thistle into a large pot with 2 quarts of water and 2 pints of moonshine. Set to medium-high heat and let boil until it thickens.[19]

Step 2: Pour all 10 gallons of store-bought potato soup into a cauldron big enough to hold it, and bring to a simmer.

Step 3: Once simmering, add 3 pints of moonshine, all of the butter, all of the black pepper, and bring to a boil.

Step 4: When it comes to a boil, lower the temperature to simmer and add the milk thistle; stir vigorously with the end of a broomstick.

Step 5: Serve it up with crackers, bread, or something else that will help kill the taste.

Cassy's Carrot Cake

This recipe is the camp favorite! Ranch hands, campers, even Sheriff Buck Mueller come running to the ranch house to get a slice. This carrot cake has been known to sustain Shari Running Wild for weeks while she roamed the countryside attacking settlers.

Cake

Ingredients:

      1 cup oil
      2 cups shredded baby carrots (shred
      them in the food processor)
      2 cups sugar
      1 can crushed pineapple (in its own juice)
      3 eggs
      2 teaspoons of cinnamon
      2 teaspoons baking soda
      1 teaspoon salt

---

[19] If you are Mormon, Muslim, or belong to another non-alcoholic consuming religion, don't fret; Cookie hasn't realized that all of the alcohol burns off in the cooking process!

    1 cup sweetened coconut flakes
    2 cups flour
    1 cup pecan pieces

Step 1: Mix all ingredients well.
Step 2: Bake in two 8 1/2 inch diameter by 1 5/16 inch pans at 350
    degrees for 45 minutes.

Icing

Ingredients:

    Pre-made cream cheese frosting
    1 teaspoon vanilla
    1 cup sweetened coconut flakes
    1 cup pecans (finely chopped)

Step 1. Toast coconut in oven to desired color
Step 2. Heat frosting in microwave 10–15 seconds (remove top and
    aluminum cover first)
Step 3. Mix well with vanilla
Step 4. Apply to cake and sprinkle with the toasted coconut and nuts

Cookie's Medicinal Moonshine

Menard County's' favorite illegal contraband is Cookie's moonshine. This dangerous liquid provides the means to leave reality for a while, then it will return with an enormous throbbing headache! This recipe creates about 5 gallons of the wonderful brew.

Ingredients:

    5 gallons wash water
    7 lbs cracked corn
    7 lbs of granulated sugar
    1 tbsp yeast

Step 1: Find a remote location where the feds won't find you and set up your still.

Step 2: Put your ingredients into the fermenter in the order listed and close it. Fermentation of the sugar will begin in about 12 hours. It will take 3 or 4 days for the ebullition to end, at which time you can siphon your beer out of the fermenter with a racking cane and charge your still.

Step 3: For your first run, pot distill your wash and keep things running slowly. Periodically put 4–5 drops of distillate into a spoon with an equal amount of water and taste it to identify the off-taste of the heads.

Step 4: For your second fermentation, the fermenter should have 3–3/4 gallons of water; to include your old barm and corn, take 1–1/4 gallons of backset from your first distillation and add another 7 pounds of granulated sugar. Then add this mixture of sugar and cooled backset to the fermenter, which should contain 3–3/4 gallons of water. This will bring your total beer volume back to 5 gallons. Now remove the spent corn kernels floating on top of the fermenter and replace with new cracked corn.

Step 5: For the second run, siphon off the beer and charge your still by replacing 3–3/4 gallons of water into the fermenter so the yeast doesn't die. Distill your whiskey the same way you did during the first run.

Now you have great medicinal white lightning!

Possum on a Stick (a campfire treat!)

Campers usually enjoyed this treat until the ingredients are known, so keep it a secret until all has been consumed.

Ingredients:

    10 baby possums—skinned and cleaned
    with the heads and tails removed.

10 long live oak tree sticks, approximately 1/2
inch in diameter and at least 5 feet in length.
A good campfire, burned down to a
low flame, with lots of hot coals.

Step 1: Send someone out to the wilderness to collect baby possums;
its best that you find someone like Cassy who knows the way
of the possum.
Step 2: Skewer the possum lengthwise, do not skewer through the
middle as they may fall into the fire while cooking.
Step 3: Rotate the possums slowly over the open fire until the grease
stops surfacing. It should take approximately 7 minutes over a
hot fire, or 10 minutes over a low fire. Make sure your sticks do
not catch fire as they will burn rapidly!

Now sit back and eat a treat!

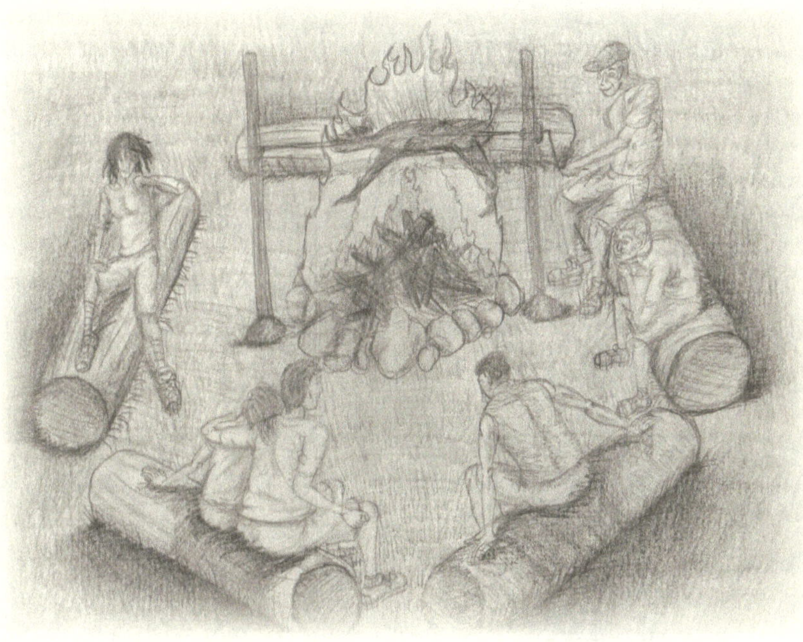

Fried Rattlesnake (or any snake for that matter)

Some say rattlesnake tastes like chicken, but it doesn't, it tastes like snake. We have a variety of snakes on PSL Ranch, but the rattler is the largest and easiest to find as they tend to *rattle* when you get close to them!

Ingredients:

> 4–6-foot rattle snake, skinned and cleaned.
> 2 eggs
> 1/4 cup whole milk
> Teaspoon of salt
> Teaspoon of black pepper
> 2 cups of cooking oil or lard
> 1 cup of flour

Step 1: Find a snake. If you are not certain how to catch a rattlesnake, drive around the county roads and look for a fresh kill. To determine if the snake died recently, look to see if it is still wiggling, or look for buzzards trying to eat one. Buzzards only eat fresh meat.

Step 2: Cut the head off and leave it—a dead snake can still inject poison if you are not careful.

Step 3: Skin, clean, and wash the meat, cutting it into 4 inch lengths.

Step 4: Add the eggs and milk into a mixing bowl and beat until smooth.

Step 5: Mix the salt, pepper, and flour into a bowl.

Step 6: Preheat a frying pan with the oil or lard.

Step 7: Dip the snake pieces into the egg mixture and then into the flour and spices, placing it into the hot oil.

Step 8: Cook until golden brown.

There you have it! If you don't want to fight with bones, just use the back meat. It will be a little stringy, but will satisfy the most discerning pallet!

Cookie's Dead Critter Stew

So you found something dead and it hasn't started stinking. Why waste nature's gift! PSL Ranch wants your camping experience to be one with nature while at the same time saving money on expensive store-bought meat! It's easy to find dead critters as they are littered alongside the road, from deer to buzzards, and they are all good eating! To identify edible meat, look for buzzards enjoying a snack, they only eat fresh meat so it's sure to be good! We suggest cutting away the part of the critter that was struck by the passing vehicle.

Ingredients for 10 servings:

> 8 pounds of critter meat
> 1 cup of flour
> 2 tablespoon of salt
> 2 tablespoon of pepper
> Garlic, Paprika, and Bay leaf (to taste)
> Worcestershire sauce
> 1 large onion
> 5 large potatoes
> 2 large carrots
> 2 large celery stalks

Step 1: Skin, gut, and clean dead critter, making sure you cut away damaged areas and parts the buzzards were eating.
Step 2: Cut meat into 1-inch cubes and place in a large cooking pot.
Step 3: In a medium-sized bowl, mix the flour, salt, and pepper; pour over meat, stirring to coat the meat with the flour and spices.
Step 4: Slowly stir in the garlic, bay leaf, paprika, and Worcestershire sauce; amounts vary on taste and preference.
Step 5: Chop and add in onion, potatoes, carrots, and celery, stirring to ensure even distribution.
Step 6: Cover and cook on low for 10 to 12 hours. Serve hot!

There you have it, a feast for 10 for only a few dollars! Your guests will never know what they are eating and will enjoy every bite.

Cassy's Saint Jago Pork Chops

This recipe has been handed down through the generations from Cassy's Jamaican ancestors and is devoured by the ranch hands! It takes a while, but is well worth it and serves 4 (we don't give this to the campers)!

Ingredients:

> 2 pounds trimmed pork chops (*do not* substitute skunk or possum meat!)
> 1 cup tomato ketchup
> 2 cups water
> 1 tablespoon pepper
> 1 tablespoon salt
> 1 cup white flour
> 1 teaspoon lard or vegetable oil
> 3 teaspoon soy sauce
> 1 small onion—chopped

Step 1: Brown onions in lard in large frying pan; remove and put in shallow baking dish
Step 2: Dredge chops in flour and brown in large frying pan
Step 3: Add salt, pepper, and water to pan, and bring to a boil
Step 4: Place chops in shallow baking dish and add liquid
Step 5: Cover and cook for 45 minutes at 350 degrees
Step 6: Mix ketchup and soy sauce in small mixing bowl
Step 7: Remove foil or cover, and add the ketchup-soy sauce mixture to top of each chop, and mix rest into the liquid; cook uncovered for 15 more minutes

Cassy suggests serving this dish hot on a bed of white rice with your favorite salad dish!

Cookie's Possum Tail Omelet (with or without cheese)

Some of you may be thinking, what happened to the mother of those poor baby possums used in our Possum on a Stick recipe? Well, she didn't go to waste! The body is conveniently used in Cookie's Dead Critter Stew and the tails make a great omelet, so read on and prepare for a treat! This recipe feeds ten hungry campers

Ingredients:

      1/2 pound of salted butter
      2 dozen eggs
      1 cup cream or heavy cream
      1 tablespoon of salt
      1 tablespoon of black pepper
      5 adult possum tails (raccoon
      tails can be substituted)
      Shredded cheddar cheese (optional)

Step 1: Add eggs (without shells) into a large mixing bowl and add cream.

Step 2: Add salt and pepper, and mix thoroughly until the mixture is smooth.

Step 3: Cut cleaned-and-washed possum tails in 1/2 inch circular pieces, being careful to stop 2 inches from the end, as it is too small.

Step 4: Add possum tail pieces to egg mixture and stir until evenly distributed.

Step 5: Melt butter in large frying pan (2 pans may be necessary) and add omelet mixture.

Step 6: Cook until mixture is golden brown, flipping on occasion. Serve immediately.

Step 7: Sprinkle shredded cheese over top of omelet if desired.

Wow, what a breakfast! You may want to warn your guests that there are little bones in their omelets so they don't choke and die.

Also, if you want to use fresh possum tails, make sure you hold the possum by the scruff of the neck when chopping their tails off —if they're just playing dead this may rouse them!

Slim's Famous BBQ

Slim is well known for his brisket barbeque, and we now have his secret! This meal can serve any number of guests; just let him know how many need to be fed three hours before mealtime!

Ingredients:

> At least 1/4 tank of gas in Slim's old truck
> A PSL Ranch credit card
> Cell connectivity
> A cooler to keep food warm

Step 1: Identify how many have to be fed.

Step 2: one-and-a-half hours prior to meal time, climb into Slim's old truck and head towards Junction, Texas, approximately a forty-minute drive from PSL Ranch.

Step 3: While driving through Menard, call Coopie's BBQ in Junction and put in an order for the appropriate amount of brisket required for the meal.

Step 4: *Do not* stop at Uncle Weirdo's Tavern for a beer!

Step 5: Once at Coopie's Bar-B-Q & Grill, use PSL Ranch's credit card to pay for the meal, and place brisket into cooler to keep warm.

Step 6: Drive the speed limit back to PSL Ranch as there are always state troopers and sheriff's deputies along the way.

Step 7: *Do not* stop at Uncle Weirdo's Tavern for a beer!

Step 8: Go through the backdoor of the ranch house with cooler and transfer meat to a large roaster. Place roaster in oven at 200 degrees and call everyone in for dinner.

There you go! Your guests will marvel at the quality of your brisket and no one knows the better!

Cookie's Scrambled Eggs (Vulture, Turkey, or Chicken)

While strolling around PSL Ranch, you might come across a batch of turkey eggs, or a couple of vulture eggs that fell out of a tree when a bull snake tried to eat them. If you're really lucky, someone may have stolen a batch of fresh chicken eggs from a local farmer. In any case, Cookie knows how to cook up a great batch of scrambled eggs.

Ingredients:

> 6 turkey eggs, or 4 buzzard eggs, or 1 dozen
> chicken eggs. If using turkey or buzzard eggs,
> look to see if they are green when broken
> 1/2 pound of salted butter
> 1/2 cup of cream or heavy cream
> 1 tablespoon of salt
> 1 tablespoon of black pepper

Step 1: Add eggs without the shells into a large mixing bowl.
Step 2: Add pepper, salt, and cream; mixing to a smooth consistency.
Step 3: Melt butter in a large frying pan until bubbling.
Step 4: Add egg mixture and occasionally mix until they appear dry with a little browning. For runny eggs, cook less, but if the eggs were green when broken, cook until dry to reduce the chance of food poisoning.

That's all there is to it! Now you have creamy and buttery eggs that will warm your stomach!

Cassy's Crockpot Chili

Another ranch hand favorite not shared with the campers is Cassy's secret Crockpot Chili, the best we've ever tasted! This Jamaican version of Texas Chili includes a taste of the Caribbean that can't be beat, and it won't make you toot. Cassy would be mighty angry if she knew we were giving this one away!

Ingredients for 4 heaping helpings:

> 2 pound ground beef
> 2 medium onions, chopped
> 1/4 teaspoon dried garlic pieces
> 1 can (16 ounce) pinto or red kidney beans
> 1 can (15 ounce) stewed tomatoes, chopped
> 1 teaspoon salt
> 2–3 tablespoons chili powder
> 2 tablespoons curry powder
> (Use a 1000-watt microwave or
> adjust time accordingly)

Step 1: Crumble ground beef in 3-quart casserole bowl.
Step 2: Stir in onion and garlic.
Step 3: Cook at high for 6 to 7 minutes, stir once and drain.
Step 4: Stir in remaining ingredients.
Step 5: Cover with lid and cook at high for 7 minutes.
Step 6: Continue cooking at medium-low for 35–40 minutes; stir occasionally.
Step 7: Stir, then let stand covered for 7 minutes before serving.

This is far too good for campers, so keep it to yourself and eat alone!!

Cookie's Spicy Skunk Soup

Most people think you can't eat a skunk, but they don't know what they're missing! Cookie's recipe was concocted during a slow period in which business wasn't very good and deer season was still a way off. So if you're on a budget and spot a skunk, this one is for you! One healthy skunk feeds four.

Ingredients:

> 1 healthy skunk, approximately 3 pounds when
> cleaned and gutted, or two sickly skunks.
> One gallon of beef broth (chicken broth
> can be substituted for a lighter taste).
> Parsley (to taste)
> 2 tablespoons of salt
> 4 tablespoons of black pepper
> 4 clothesline pins

Step 1: Debone the skunk and cut into 1/2 inch pieces. We strongly recommend using a face mask or use some other way to decrease the stench while preparing.

Step 2: Add beef broth, salt, pepper, parsley, and skunk chunks into large pot.

Step 3: Bring to a boil and let simmer for 2 hours.

Step 4: Provide a clothesline pin for each guest and serve hot!

Some diners prefer hot sauce to add some additional spice and flavor, but most just use clothespins to kill the smell as they eat. Enjoy!

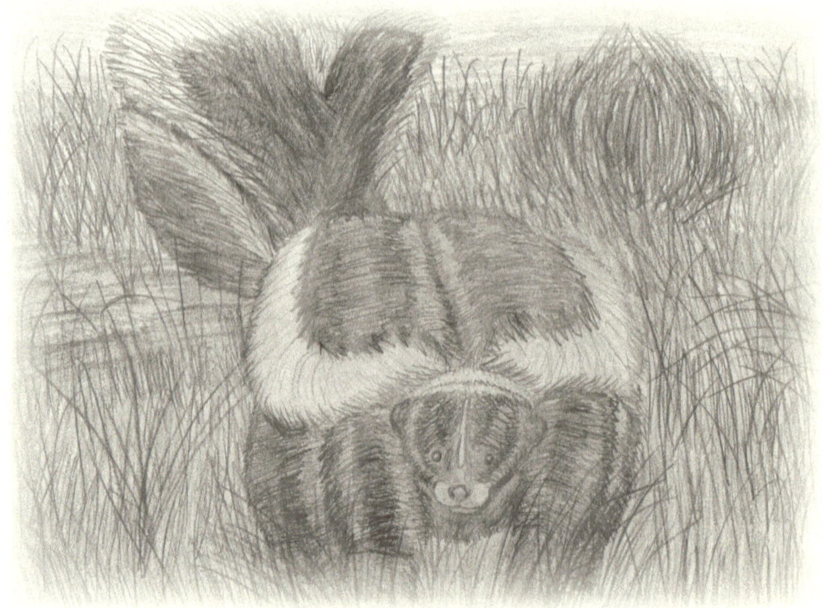

Cassy's Bread Pudding and Whiskey Sauce

This recipe was stolen from a rival ranch after an innocent visit by Cassy, Slim, Dr. S, and Shari Running Wild many years ago. Cassy begged for the recipe and with the help of a little black magic, was able to learn everything from their cook except how to make the whiskey sauce. After many years of trying multiple whiskeys and cream recipes, Cassy finally found it. Now it's yours!

Ingredients:

> 2 cups bread cubes (use white bread
> for best taste and texture)
> 2 cups whole milk
> 3 tablespoon butter (melted)
> 1/4 cup sugar
> 2 eggs slightly beaten
> 1/2 teaspoon vanilla
> Dash of salt

Step 1: Place bread cubes in buttered 1-quart baking dish.
Step 2: Scald milk; stir in butter and sugar.
Step 3: Mix eggs, vanilla, and salt; pour over bread cubes.
Step 4: Set baking dish in larger baking pan. Fill outer pan with water up to the level of the pudding.
Step 5: Bake at 350 degrees for 60–65 minutes, or until knife inserted in middle of pudding comes out clean.

Cassy suggests serving with her famous whiskey sauce, made as follows:

Step 1. Take one can condensed milk and heat on low in small sauce pan.
Step 2. Add 1 shot of Texas whiskey and stir (drink 2 shots as you deserve it).
Now pour the whiskey sauce over the bread pudding and enjoy!

Cassy's Homemade Flapjacks

These ain't no ordinary flapjacks, and should be made on those mornings when you want something extra for your breakfast! Made from an old family recipe, Cassy adds a little something extra to give them their one-of-a-kind taste! Best served with a slab of bacon and some fresh cooked eggs!

Ingredients:

2 cups flour
3 teaspoons baking powder
1/2 teaspoon salt
3 eggs—separated
1 3/4 cups buttermilk
4 tablespoons butter (melted)
3 tablespoons sugar

Step 1: Combine the flour, baking powder, and salt in a bowl.
Step 2: In a separate bowl, beat the egg yolks, then add the butter-milk and butter, and stir to blend.
Step 3: Combine the flour and yolk mixture, and beat until smooth.
Step 4: Beat the egg whites until stiff—but not dry.
Step 5: Slowly add the sugar while beating constantly.
Step 6: Mix a third of the beaten whites gently into the batter, then fold in the remaining whites very carefully.
Step 7: Add 1 teaspoon of almond extract, or to taste.
Step 7: Spread 1/2 cup of the batter onto a hot griddle and flip when bubbling. Cook until golden brown.

We're not sure why, but the thing about this recipe Cassy likes most is beaten them whites! We sure hope you enjoy these extra-light and tasty breakfast treats.

Jamaican Patois to English Translations

To make it easier for campers and other visitors to understand Cassy, and to avoid another incident like #23, PSL Ranch has provided basic translations for words and sayings often used by Cassy when instructing campers around the ranch house. They are not listed in alphabetical order; rather, they are listed by how frequently Cassy uses them. We feel this will help make your stay more enjoyable, and less lethal.

If mi catch u pon di couch wit u dutty clothes, u dead!: Take off your dirty clothes before sitting on my couch

If mi catch u inna mi ouse wit u dutty shoes, u dead!: Take off your dirty shoes before entering my cabin

Dat is paison… u mad?: You shouldn't eat that, it's poisonous.

Nu mek faiya catch u… lef it alone!: You shouldn't touch that, it burns!

Nu trouble dat, it naa trouble u: You shouldn't pet that, it's dangerous.

Yu nu see di foam inna it mout… run fah yu life! You shouldn't pet that; it has rabies!

Yu nu see it cole out ear. Put on yu jacket!: You should dress warmer, it's cold outside!

Yu waa get eat stroke? Tek off some a yu clothes!: You shouldn't dress so warm, it's hot outside!

Yu betta tek more wahta dan dat!: You'd better take enough water for your hike!

Nuh leave nuh mess n ear… mi not yu madda!: Clean up after yourself!

Pig is food, not fren!: Pigs are for shooting and eating, not playing with!

Mine yuself… cow will run yu down!: The cattle are not tame!

Nu touch dat… it will ot yu!: You shouldn't touch that, it'll hurt!

Yu nah go outside, stahm adeh: Don't go outside, there's a tornado.

Keep uself still… yu wha ice conk yu inna yu ead?: Don't go outside, it's hailing.

Keep uself still… nu mek lightning kech yu!: Don't go outside, there's severe lightning!

Dat wahta a go drown yu!: Stay out of the lake!

Laad God! Faiya inna di wood! Run, mi se run!: It's a wildfire, run!

Pickney: Child.

Pickney dem: Children.

Yu eat Cookie food, yu ded: Cookie's cooking will kill you.

Puhs: Cat (large or small).

Tupid pickney: Stupid child.

Mi se gwaan: Get away from me.

Nuh bahda mi: Don't bother me.

Laad a maasy! Mek mi ears eat grass!: Stop talking!

Drop di gun pickney! Yu waa kill sumody: Put that gun down child!

If yu shoot di arrow inna di sky, it acome lik yu inna yu eye!: Don't shoot arrows straight up!

Wat a ugly pickney!: you're an ugly child!

Edback: Back of the head.

Fahrid: Front of the head.

Ooh tink up di place?: Who farted?

Aneda one: Another one.

Awho dat?: Who is that?

Awha dat?: What is that?

Awhe yu go?: Where are you going?

Dis ting kya fix?: Is it broken?

No bahda mi!: Leave me alone!

Green Tree Campers of America Sponsors

The cost of sending hundreds of GTCA campers to PSL Ranch so they may experience the great Central Texas outdoors can be overwhelming for some families. To help defray costs, the following sponsors provide financial assistance at a low interest rate to campers who can't afford the trip on their own. Please take time to look at our GTCA sponsors and send them an email of appreciation!

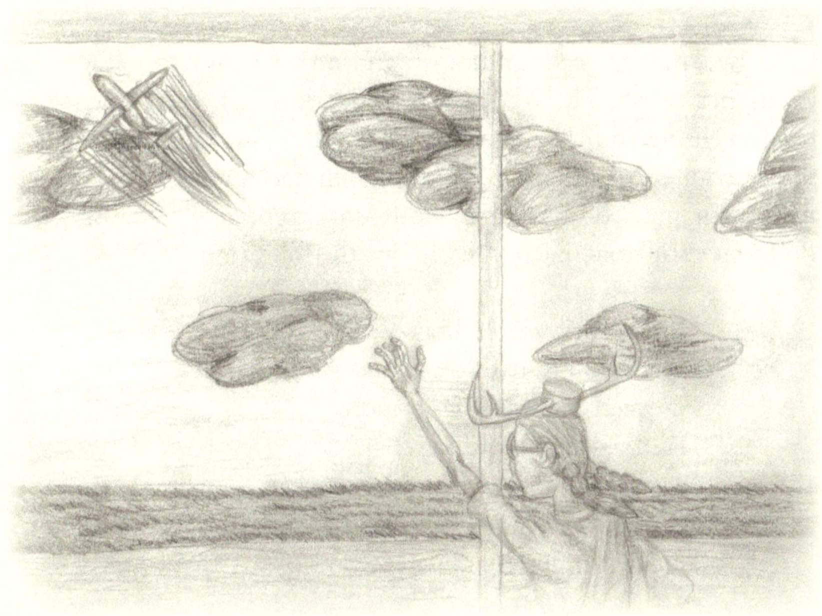

GTCA Gold Sponsor: Kitty-B-Gone

Give your dead kitty, or one that's on its way, a proper cremation with little or no pain with:

Kitty-B-Gone Self-Help Cremation Kit

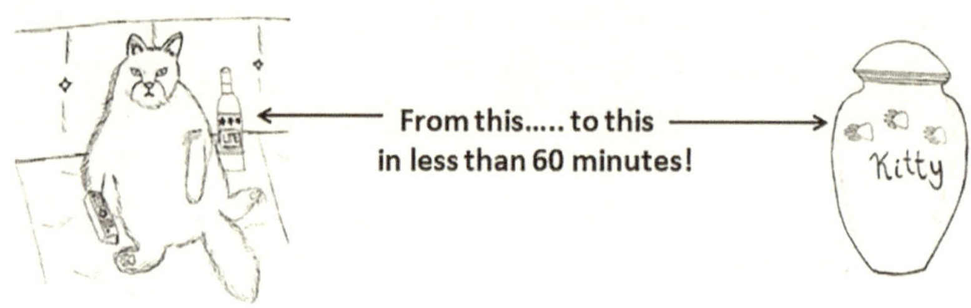

Awe, puss is dead, or almost, and now it's time to reduce your loving pet to ash. The KBG kit provides you with everything you'll need to ensure your pet puss used its last life. Our kit includes everything required to sustain a fire at the temperature necessary to cremate your puss, or at least make it unrecognizable to those pesky PETA investigators. Each kit contains the following:

- One cat urn, small, brass
- Lighter Fluid, twelve ounces
- Fourteen-inch slip-knot noose
- Gallon-sized plastic bag
- Mayan End-of-Days ignition sticks
- Wooden noseclip
- Small hammer

Visit our website for more exciting products, to include our Award-winning Grandma-B-Gone!

GTCA Silver Sponsor: Menard Mortuary and Barbershop

Visit Menard Mortuary and Barbershop and get the service you deserve from Dan Parkinson. Whether it's a casket made of the finest mesquite, or a plot to put it in, Dan is your man! With over 70 years of experience, you can also enjoy a fancy haircut by this sure-handed barber while you wait for your loved one to be eternally interned. Select from one of our packages for the best deal in town!

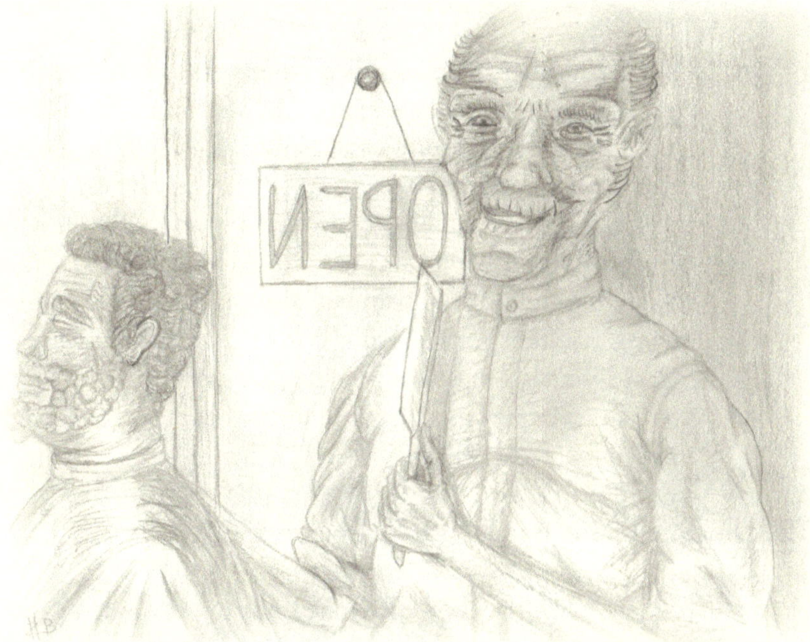

The Budget Plan: $65.00

- Select from one of three rugs to wrap your loved one in for burial. All our cloth burials include duct tape to ensure they don't slide out on their way down. Embalming, church service, grave digging, and transportation to the plot are extra.

The Real Deal: $225.00

- Our best seller, the Real Deal, includes a mesquite wood casket hand-made by Dan to fit any stiff! Dan will make sure your loved one gets a proper send-off to include transportation to the gravesite and a sentimental reading to include the bible verse of your choice. Embalming and grave digging are extra.

The All-inclusive Plan: $375.00

- Our premium plan takes all of the work out of sending your loved one to a better place, and we don't mean Brady! Dan provides a mesquite casket and will even plug all the holes so no body parts hang out. He embalms the stiff using Cookie's embalming fluid and any leftover fluid will be passed around to mourners during services to alleviate any feelings of sadness. Dan will also make sure your loved one's gravesite is properly dug in the correct location and marked with a limestone boulder. This plan also includes up to three bible verses that will be read with real feeling to make it seem like we care.

The Ultimate Viking Burial on Lake Rohret: $750.00

- Imagine your loved one stretched out on a wooden canoe made to look like a Viking ship and set sail across Lake Rohret. Doused with gas, Shari Running Wild will shoot a flaming arrow into the craft once it reaches a depth of three feet or more. You can enjoy home brew as your loved one turns to ash and slowly sinks into Valhalla! This funeral experience is by far our most enjoyable, but is dependent on weather, specifically, torrential rains.

For more information call: 742-594-2637 or email parkinsons@shaky.com.

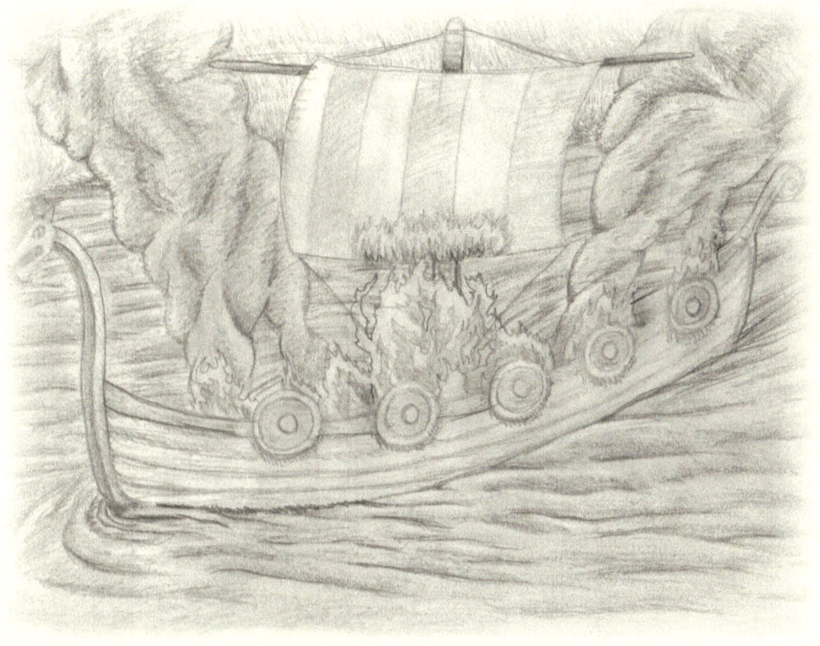

GTCA Bronze Sponsor: Menard
Grave Diggers Association

MGDA is proud to sponsor GTCA campers at PSL Ranch. If you need some grave digging, and can't do it yourself, contact MGDA Local 666 and we'll provide you a list of qualified Union diggers that will proudly dig your hole.

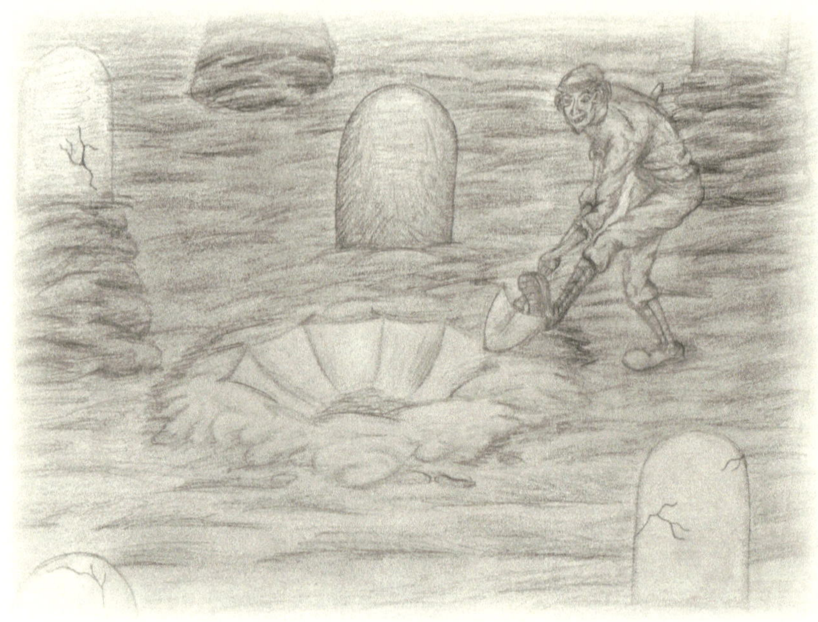

For digging services, call 1-800-344-3337, or email, sixfeet-deep@mgda.com.

About Our Illustrator
Sketch

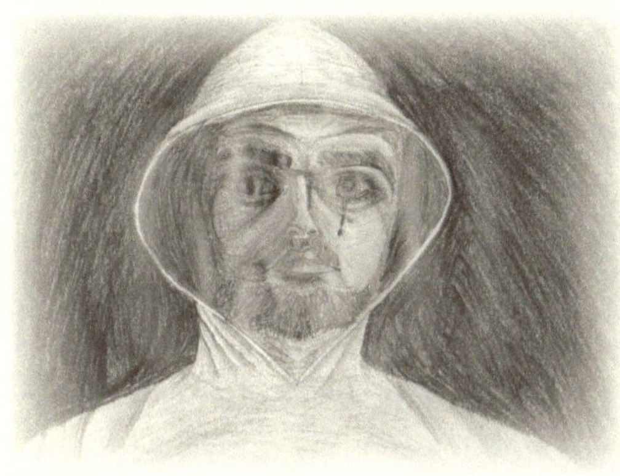

At the beginning of this project, the authors decided that illustrations would enhance the information provided as well as making it a more enjoyable read! In searching for the right individual to accomplish the chore of illustrating such an important document, we visited multiple businesses that said they were up to the task. After reviewing their quotes, we began looking for starving artists under some of the most prestigious overpasses between San Angelo and San Antonio, and that's where we met Sketch; a local artist of questionable origin. Sketch was wearing tattered clothing and a hoodie, supporting a fake eye patch as he limped through the vehicles at a stoplight with a sign that read, "Will Sketch for Food." One of the authors noticed a high-quality drawing in a corner of his sign showing a young man in a straitjacket (obviously a self-portrait). Though his methods were questionable, he impressed PSL with some of his previous work to include many portraits of people, some of whom we're even aware of the fact (though most were drawn encased in a window). After careful review, we immediately hired Sketch! Little is known about him since he usually delivered his sketches by leaving a portfolio of artwork near specified bus stops, but fifty-seven Big Mac meals later (most were supersized—we spared no expense) our safety guide was adorned with his work!

For more information about Sketch, visit www.whatkilledsally.com/sketch, or call the San Antonio Police Department for his files.

PSL Store Items

www.whatkilledsally.com/store

PSL staff and ranch hands are frequently asked is we have any products that can be purchased online, or that can be acquired through the Dark Web. Well of course we do! Check out a few of the items below, but remember, prices do not include shipping or fines for shipping contraband via USPS.

Item	Description	Cost	Additional Info
PSL001	Cow Chips (dry)	$25.00	Varying sizes— same price
PSL002	Cow Pies (wet)	$50.00	Try standing behind a cow!
PSL003	Natural wood Coasters	$30.00	May be uneven and wobble
PSL004	PSL Cookbook	100.00	In progress, but you can pay now
PSL005	Indian Headband	$250.00	Customized by Shari Running Wild
PSL006	Ancient Alien Rock Carvings	$300.00	May appear like their new!
PSL007	Original PSL T-shirt	$25.00	High quality cotton
PSL008	Chert	$15.00	For making arrow heads
PSL009	PSL Calendar	$17.50	Using our own artwork!

PSL010	What Killed Sally Updates	$20.00	Monthly update via USPS
PSL011	Piece of PSL cactus	$10.00	Thorns included
PSL012	What Killed Sally	$35.00	Signed copy with inscription
PSL013	Teaspoon of Cocoa's ashes	$250.00	While supplies last
PSL014	Pint of Cow Dung Dew	$225.00	Cookies best (attempt)
PSL015	Mobile Safe Place	$500.00	Comes with sound dampeners

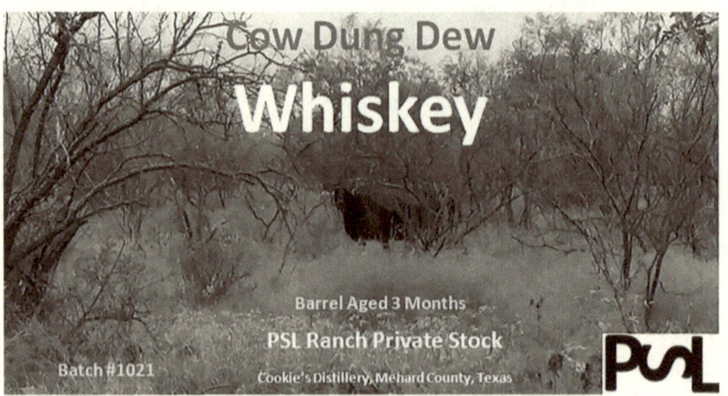

Guaranteed to make anybody look better
after 3 shots, or your money back[20]

---

[20] Warning: Results may vary due to individual liver function and eye health. Guarantee is void if customer is blind or is a hardened alcoholic, also known as Cookie's syndrome. Millennials are advised to drink several Shirley Temples and find a safe space before partaking in this fine beverage.

Look at what others have said after reading *What Killed Sally?*

What? Get the hell off the phone!
—FBI

(When called to comment about the accuracy of the
bureau's investigations into Sally's demise)

Kick up Rumpus.
—Jamaican Tourist Council

If she could read, I'm sure Congresswoman
Waters would not like this book.
—Random Drug Addict

I've read all the Sally books—*Sally at the Farm, Sally in
the Snow, Sally in the Forest, Silly Sally,* and of course
the classic, *Harry became Sally*—but it wasn't until
I read *What Killed Sally* did it all make sense!
—Anonymous recent ex-President

About the Author

Slim is a computer scientist and a distinguished engineer with a passion for the outdoors. Raised on a farm in Iowa, he now resides in Texas with his beautiful and very independent Jamaican American wife. Slim has published and presented over twenty-five technical papers, and *What Killed Sally* was written with the same dedication to detail and accuracy as the rest of his works. With over thirty-four years of experience working with government contracts and personnel, his view of the world has assuredly been affected!